Atlantis Ambient and Pervasive Intelligence

Volume 8

Series Editor

Ismail Khalil, Johannes Kepler University, Linz, Austria

For further volumes:
www.atlantis-press.com

Aims and Scope of the Series

The book series 'Atlantis Ambient and Pervasive Intelligence' publishes high quality titles in the fields of Pervasive Computing, Mixed Reality, Wearable Computing, Location-Aware Computing, Ambient Interfaces, Tangible Interfaces, Smart Environments, Intelligent Interfaces, Software Agents and other related fields. We welcome submission of book proposals from researchers worldwide who aim at sharing their results in this important research area.

For more information on this series and our other book series, please visit our website at:

www.atlantis-press.com/publications/books
Atlantis Press
29, avenue Laumière
75019 Paris, France

Tibor Bosse · Diane J. Cook
Mark Neerincx · Fariba Sadri
Editors

Human Aspects in Ambient Intelligence

Contemporary Challenges and Solutions

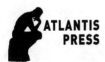
ATLANTIS
PRESS

Editors

Tibor Bosse
Department of Computer Science
VU University Amsterdam
Amsterdam
The Netherlands

Diane J. Cook
School of Electrical Engineering
  and Computer Science
Washington State University
Pullman, WA
USA

Mark Neerincx
Department of Intelligent Systems
Delft University of Technology
Delft
The Netherlands

Fariba Sadri
Department of Computing
Imperial College London
London
UK

ISSN 1875-7669
ISBN 978-94-6239-017-1   ISBN 978-94-6239-018-8   (eBook)
DOI 10.2991/978-94-6239-018-8

Library of Congress Control Number: 2013947571

Printed on acid-free paper

Preface

Since the late 1990s, Ambient Intelligence (AmI) has been put forward as a vision on the near future of computing. As such, it refers to a world in which human beings are surrounded by intelligent electronic systems that are unobtrusively incorporated in their environment, monitor their behavior using sensors, and support them in their daily activities. Based on this definition, a book on *Human Aspects in Ambient Intelligence* may appear a bit tautological at first sight. After all, the word 'ambient' comes from the Latin verb 'ambire', which literally means 'to go around' or 'to surround.' And following the AmI perspective, the objects that are 'surrounded'—by intelligent technology in this case—are human beings. Hence, would not any book on AmI automatically address human aspects?

Although this sounds like a logical line of reasoning, it is not entirely true. First, AmI is a very broad, multidisciplinary field of study, which also includes various technical ingredients that are not necessarily related to humans, such as distributed computing, embedded systems, and sensor fusion. Second, rather than addressing human aspects in general, the current book has a specific focus on AmI systems that *understand* humans. The underlying assumption is that AmI systems that exploit *knowledge about human functioning* are better equipped to understand the needs of human beings, enabling them to provide more adequate and personalized support. To realize such knowledgeable AmI systems, a variety of elements is required, including theories from the human-directed sciences (e.g., psychology, social sciences, neurosciences, and biomedical sciences) as well as techniques to apply the appropriate knowledge in an intelligent manner (e.g., knowledge representation and reasoning, agent technology, and machine learning).

Hence, the current book can be distinguished from other AmI books due to its emphasis on AmI systems that provide knowledgeable support, based on detailed analyses on human states and processes. This book comprises 10 chapters, most of which are improved and extended versions of papers presented at the Sixth International Workshop on *Human Aspects in Ambient Intelligence*, which was held in November 2012 in Pisa, Italy, as part of the International Joint Conference on Ambient Intelligence. In addition, this book contains three invited chapters, written by international experts in the field. The material of each chapter is self-contained and was reviewed by at least two anonymous referees, to assure a high quality. Readers can select any individual chapter based on their research interests, without the need of reading other chapters. As a consequence, there is no straightforward order in which the different chapters should be presented. Nevertheless, in an attempt to create some structure, the 10 chapters have been clustered into four parts, which can be described as follows:

Part I: Mental State Analysis
Part II: Motion Tracking
Part III: Lifestyle Support
Part IV: mHealth Applications

Note that Part I and II have an emphasis on *analysis* of human aspects, whereas Part III and IV focus on *support* of humans based on such analyses.

In particular, the first part contains two chapters that present approaches to analyze mental states of humans, especially intentions (Sadri et al.) and trust states (Toubman et al.), which can be used to develop more personalized AmI systems.

The second part comprises three chapters that illustrate how AmI systems may benefit from analyses of human behavior based on motion (and related) sensors. These include methods to assess human beings' nonverbal expressive and emotional behavior (Piana et al.), to identify residents of smart homes through their behavior (Crandall and Cook), and to build acoustic maps of a human's spatial environment (Scattolin et al.).

The third part consists of three chapters that introduce agent-based AmI systems to support human beings in adopting a suitable lifestyle. The systems described in this part involve personal coaches to support people in learning movement patterns (Bobbert et al.), virtual coaches to assist people in changing lifestyles (Roelofsma and Kurt), and an agent-based architecture to manage energy consumption (Zupančič et al.).

The fourth and last part of this book is composed of two chapters that apply the AmI paradigm to mobile health applications. These chapters address, respectively, an approach to adapt mobile (healthcare) services intelligently to the user's needs (Wac and Ullah), and a mobile phone application to help people manage life-threatening allergies (Hernandez-Munoz and Woolley).

We are confident that this combination of chapters provides useful reference values to researchers and students with an interest in human aspects of AmI, enabling them to find solutions and recognize challenges in the field.

To conclude, we wish to express our gratitude to all who contributed to the publication of this book, including all authors for sharing their interesting research with us, all reviewers for guarding the quality of the chapters, and last but not least, to the series editor and the publisher of the Atlantis Ambient and Pervasive Intelligence book series for offering us the opportunity to publish this volume.

Tibor Bosse
Diane J. Cook
Mark Neerincx
Fariba Sadri

Contents

Part I
Mental State Analysis

Chapter 1
A Clustering Approach to Intention Recognition

Fariba Sadri, Weikun Wang and Afroditi Xafi

Intention recognition has significant applications in ambient intelligence, assisted living and care of the elderly, games and intrusion and other crime detection. In this chapter we explore an approach to intention recognition based on clustering. To this end we show how to map the intention recognition problem into a clustering problem. We then use three different clustering algorithms, Fuzzy C-means, Possibilistic C-means and Improved Possibilistic C-means. We illustrate and compare their effectiveness empirically using a variety of test cases, including cases involving noisy or partial data. To our knowledge the use of clustering techniques for intention recognition is novel, and this chapter suggests it is promising.

1.1 Introduction

Intention recognition (IR) is the problem of recognising the intentions[1] of an agent by (incrementally) observing its actions. Plan recognition goes further than intention recognition, and additionally attempts to recognise the plan (sequence of actions, including some not yet observed) the observed agent is pursuing. Many applications of intention recognition have been explored, including Unix-based help facilities and story understanding, in its earlier years, and ambient intelligence, elder care,

---

[1] In this chapter we use intention and goal synonymously.

F. Sadri (✉) · W. Wang · A. Xafi
Department of Computing, Imperial College London,
180 Queens Gate, London SW7 2AZ, UK
e-mail: fs@doc.ic.ac.uk

W. Wang
e-mail: ww2210@doc.ic.ac.uk

A. Xafi
e-mail: ax10@doc.ic.ac.uk

T. Bosse et al. (eds.), *Human Aspects in Ambient Intelligence*,
Atlantis Ambient and Pervasive Intelligence 8, DOI: 10.2991/978-94-6239-018-8_1,
© Atlantis Press and the authors 2013

e.g. [11, 20, 21], computer games, e.g. [5], prediction of military maneuvers, e.g. [19], and criminal intent detection, e.g. [10, 14], more recently.

Ambient intelligence (AMI) environments must be capable of anticipating the needs, desires and behaviour of their inhabitants [1] in order to provide suitable support to the inhabitants. Intention recognition can make a significant contribution to AMI systems by enabling and enriching their anticipatory capabilities.

Various techniques have been used for intention recognition. The most common are logic-based [2, 8, 23], case-based [7] and probabilistic approaches [4, 11, 20].

In this chapter we explore the use of clustering techniques for intention recognition. Clustering or cluster analysis is the task of classifying objects into groups in such a way that the objects in each group are more "similar" to one another than to objects outside the group. Clustering is more commonly applied to pattern recognition, image analysis, information retrieval, and bioinformatics. To our knowledge the application of clustering to intention recognition is novel.

In order to apply cluster analysis, the intention recognition problem has to be crafted as a clustering problem. Intuitively the fundamental functionality of an IR system is to classify observed actions into intentions (and plans to achieve intentions). Thus actions "related" to one another, according to some suitable criteria, have to be grouped within clusters identifying potential intentions.

In order to map intention recognition to a clustering problem, we have to overcome several difficulties. For example clustering is usually applied to elements modeled in Euclidean spaces. Thus we must map plans and actions to a format suitable for clustering, and we must do so in a robust fashion that can deal with noisy and partial data. To this end we need to devise a measure of "relatedness" or "similarity" between actions, and we need to devise a way of interpreting the result of the clustering, to associate an intention with each cluster, and a ranking with each intention indicating its likelihood, given some observed actions.

In the following sections, after presenting separate backgrounds for intention recognition and clustering, we discuss how we can overcome the difficulties mentioned above, to build a bridge between the two fields of intention recognition and machine learning via clustering, with promising results. We show how three clustering algorithms, Fuzzy C-Means, Possibilistic C-means and Improved Possibilistic C-means, can be applied to intention recognition, and we compare them empirically.

1.2 Background

1.2.1 Intention Recognition

The input to an intention recognition system usually consists of a sequence of observed actions (actions executed by an agent whose intention is being determined), and either a plan library, providing plans for intentions, or an action theory describing the semantics of actions in terms of their pre- and post-conditions. The task of the

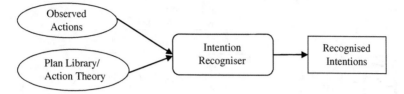

Fig. 1.1 Intention recognition

intention recognition system then is to determine the most likely goal(s) the observed agent is trying to achieve by the actions that have been observed so far and others most likely yet to be executed. This is summarised in Fig. 1.1.

Cohen et al. [6] classify intention recognition as either *intended* or *keyhole*. In the former the actor wants his intentions to be identified and intentionally gives signals to be sensed by other (observing) agents. In the latter the actor does not care whether or not his intentions are identified; he is focused on his own activities, which may provide only partial observability to other agents. This latter will be the most common case in AMI scenarios, for example in the home environment.

Intention recognition has been an active area of research for many years, and several approaches and applications have been proposed. For example, Demolombe and Fernandez [8] use logic-based specifications of macro-actions written in Golog [18], Sadri [23] and Hong [13] map reasoning about intentions with logic-based theories of causality into problems of graph generation and path finding, Geib and Goldman [11] use probabilistic techniques and plan libraries specified as Hierarchical Task Networks (HTNs), and Geib and Steedman [12] cast intention recognition as a parsing problem. They map Hierarchical Task Networks into context-free grammars, and use parsing techniques to group together individual observations into structures that are meaningful according to the grammars. A survey of the logic-based approaches can be found in [22, 24].

1.2.2 Clustering Techniques

Clustering is an unsupervised learning technique and involves the task of classifying objects into groups in such a way that the objects in each group are more "similar" to one another than to objects outside the group. Clustering involves several steps shown in Fig. 1.2. These steps will be elaborated later in the context of intention recognition.

Clustering algorithms may be *exclusive* (or hard), classifying objects into non-overlapping clusters, or *fuzzy* allowing overlapping clusters, where each object belongs to each cluster to a certain degree. They can also be *hierarchical* or *partitional*. Hierarchical approaches proceed successively by either merging smaller clusters into large ones, or by splitting large clusters into smaller ones. The end

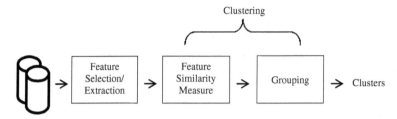

Fig. 1.2 Clustering procedure

result of the algorithm is a tree of clusters called a dendrogram, which shows the hierarchical relationship between the clusters. By cutting the dendrogram at a desired level, a clustering of the data items into groups is obtained. Partitional approaches, on the other hand, directly divide the data into a pre-determined number of clusters.

For our work we have chosen the basic C-means clustering algorithm [9] and two of its refinements [17, 26]. All three algorithms are fuzzy and partitional. These types of algorithm seem more appropriate for the application of intention recognition than hard or hierarchical types, because of the following reasons. Firstly an action may be part of a plan for achieving more than one intention, thus the suitability of fuzzy techniques. For example *getting milk from the fridge* may be an action in a plan for making tea and a plan for making porridge. Secondly, in common with all other intention recognition algorithms we assume that there is a pre-determined set of possible intentions that the algorithm can recognise, and thus the suitability of partitional clustering techniques.

The similarity measure used for clustering is dependent on the domain of the data and the feature extraction applied. For instance, when data entries are represented as points in a Euclidean space, each dimension represents a feature that has descriptive power, and the Euclidean distance can be used as a way to compare proximity of two points. If the clusters involve a sufficiently small number of dimensions they can be plotted and visualized. For example one may produce a feature space of points representing different water samples across the country. Each dimension can represent the percentage of a particular chemical in the sample. Then one may apply clustering to detect areas that share common water types.

There are cases, however, where the number of dimensions/features can be high. Then dimensionality reduction is attempted by combining or transforming features or by removing features that have less discriminatory power. A number of feature extraction techniques are available, including Principal Component Analysis [15], Isomap [25], and Laplacian Eigenmap [3].

We have chosen the Laplacian Eigenmap technique because it is efficient and popular, and, crucially, it ensures that points close to each other with respect to the chosen similarity measure will be close to each other in the low dimensional space.

1.3 The Intention Recognition Task

We focus on the task of recognising the intention(s) of a single agent and cover both the intended and keyhole cases. The agent may have multiple intentions and may be interleaving action executions in pursuit of these intentions, and may make mistakes, or the sensor data may be faulty. Moreover, the agent may miss some relevant actions, or the sensors may miss recording them. Thus the data of executed actions may be partial and imperfect. We assume we have a library of plans.

Definition 1 *Plan*
   A plan is a (non-empty) sequence of actions and is associated with an intention. In effect a plan for an intention denotes the sequence of actions the execution of which will achieve the intention. An intention may have more than one plan, an action may occur in none, one or several plans, possibly for different intentions, and an action may be repeated in a plan. Example 1 shows a simple plan library consisting of plans for three intentions.

Example 1   Intention I1: *Make Tea*   Plan 1: 1, 2, 3, 4, 5
                Intention I2: *Make Cocoa*   Plan 2: 1, 2, 6, 7, 5
                Intention I3: *Make Breakfast*   Plan 3: 1, 8, 9, 10, 11

where the numbers correspond to actions as follows:

1	2	3	4	5	6	7	8	9	10	11
Get milk	Get cup	Put tea -bag in cup	Pour boiled water in cup	Add milk to cup	Boil milk	Put cocoa in cup	Get bowl	Put cereal in bowl	Pour milk in bowl	Add sugar to bowl

We observe the actions of an agent.

Definition 2 *Observations, Partial and Noisy Observations*
Observations are sequences of actions (executed by the agent whose intention is being determined). We assume the observed actions are ground (variable-free), and, as in plans, for simplicity, we denote them by numerical identifiers.
   Observations can be *partial*, in the sense that we may not observe every action that the agent executes. Observations may be *noisy*, in two different senses. Firstly, due to sensor or action recognition faults, we may observe actions incorrectly. Secondly, the agent, due to forgetfulness or confusion may execute an action by mistake, or may execute an action towards an intention that he later abandons.

Example 2   Given the plans above, sequence S1, below, is a partial sequence of observations, S2 is noisy, and S3 is an interleaved partial sequence that goes towards achieving both intentions 1 and 3 (quite a likely sequence when one is preparing breakfast!).

$$S1 = 1; 6 \qquad S2 = 1; 2; 12; 3 \qquad S3 = 1; 2; 8; 3; 9.$$

Table 1.1 A Library of plans

Intention 1			Intention 2			Intention 3		
Plan 1	Plan 2	Plan 3	Plan 4	Plan 5	Plan 6	Plan 7	Plan 8	Plan 9
11	11	11	2	2	2	10	10	10
5	5	5	1	1	1	6	6	2
11	11	11	4	4	2	2	2	2
9	9	2	5	11	5	8	11	8
12	4	12	12	4	12	8	4	8
3	3	3	9	9	9	7	7	7

In Sect. 1.4 we report results obtained for noisy and partial observations. We have also obtained similar results for interleaved observations. But, as space is short, we ignore interleaved observations in the remainder of the chapter.

Given a set of intentions $I = \{I_1, I_2, \ldots, I_n\}$, a library L of plans for these intentions, a sequence of observed actions $A = A_1; A_2; \ldots; A_k$, the intention recognition task is to identify a subset I' of I, of the *most likely* intentions in I associated with A, according to the library L. As the sequence of observed actions grows the set of most likely intentions may change.

It may help to note that in the special (and easy) case, where we have complete and "perfect" (i.e. not noisy, partial or interleaved) observations $A_1; \ldots; A_i; A_{i+1}; \ldots; A_r; \ldots; A_s; \ldots; A_m$, then $I' = \{J_1, J_2, \ldots, J_p\}$, such that $A_1; \ldots; A_i$ is a plan for achieving J_1, $A_{i+1}; \ldots; A_r$ is a plan for achieving $J_2, \ldots$ and $A_s; \ldots; A_m$ is a plan for achieving J_p.

In the next sections we refer to a slightly more elaborate library of plans than in example 1. This library is given in Table 1.1. There are three intentions, each with three plans. The actions are represented by numerical identifiers. Thus, for example, the first plan for Intention 1 is the sequence 11; 5; 11; 9; 12; 3. These numbers are not related to example 1.

1.4 The Intention Recognition Task as a Clustering Problem

To apply clustering to intention recognition we have to follow a number of steps. First we use the information in the plan library to cluster actions that occur in plans. In order to achieve this we have to invent an appropriate similarity metric for actions. The similarity metric is used to provide a pairwise similarity matrix. To this matrix we apply the Laplacian Eigenmap technique, which will then allow us to visualise the resulting clusters and identify their prototypes (centroids). Thus we will obtain a membership matrix giving the likelihood of each intention given an observed action. Finally with each incoming observed action this membership

Fig. 1.3 Flow chart of
proposed algorithm

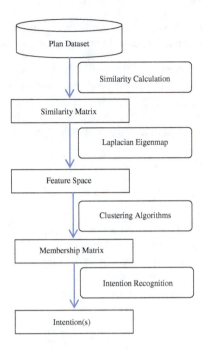

matrix is used to compute the accumulated likelihood of each intention. These steps
are summarised in Fig. 1.3.

Below we describe the main components of the algorithm.

1.4.1 Similarity Calculation for Actions

Normal similarity metrics, such as Euclidean distance and Mahalanobis distance, are
not suitable for intention recognition since we do not have a coordinate system for
actions. Instead, we propose a new similarity measure $W(i, j)$ between two actions i
and j, as follows:

$$W(i,j) = \begin{cases} \text{freq}(i,j) \frac{|P(i) \cap P(j)|}{|P(i) \cup P(j)|}, & i \neq j \\ 0, & i = j \end{cases}$$

where $P(i)$ denotes the set of plans that include action i, and $freq(i, j)$ denotes the
maximum number of times the two actions i and j occur together in any plan. The term
$freq(i, j)$ acts as a weight, so that if a pair of actions occurs many times in a plan, their
relationship (similarity) will be stronger. The term $|P(i) \cap P(j)|/|P(i) \cup P(j)|$ has
the effect that a pair of actions is similar if they co-occur in a large number of plans,
but not if either of them appears in many plans (if an action is present in many plans,
it is considered to be an untypical action). An analogy could be the prominence of

words such as "a" and "the" in the English language, and their lack of usefulness when it comes to identifying topics of a document, for example.

Example 3 The similarity between actions 3 and 5 in Table 1.1 is $W(3,5) = 0.6$. This is because the number of plans containing both actions 3 and 5 is $|P(3) \cap P(5)| = |\text{Plan1}, \text{Plan2}, \text{Plan3}| = 3$, the number of plans containing either action is $|P(3) \cup P(5)| = |\text{Plan1}, \text{Plan2}, \text{Plan3}, \text{Plan4}, \text{Plan5}, \text{Plan6}| = 5$ and the maximum frequency is freq $(3, 5) = 1$.

1.4.2 Application of Laplacian Eigenmap

After obtaining the similarity measure between pairs of actions, we use the Laplacian Eigenmap on the W matrix to extract useful and typical features from the data. The Laplacian Eigenmap technique is commonly used for clustering, and we omit the details here for lack of space. Suffice it to say that the technique solves the following minimization problem:

$$\underset{f}{\text{argmin}} \frac{1}{2} \sum_{i,j} (f_i - f_j)^2 W_{ij} = \underset{f}{\text{argmin}} \, f^T L f$$

$$f^T D f = 1$$

where D is a $|W| \times |W|$ diagonal matrix where each element is the summation of the respective column of W, $L = D-W$ is the Laplacian matrix and f is a mapping from original space W to a new space which minimises this equation. This optimisation problem is equal to solving the generalized eigenvalue problem $Lf = \lambda D f$, where λ is the eigenvalue.

These considerations can be related to the problem of intention recognition as follows. For a large value of similarity $W(i, j)$, the mapping aims to minimise the distance between i and j in the new space, which means actions i and j should be close in the new space. On the other hand, a small value of similarity $W(i, j)$ will incur a heavy penalty in the objective function, resulting in the two points being far from one another.

Example 4 Table 1.2 shows Eigenvalues 1, 2, 3 for actions 1–5, related to the plans in Table 1.1 and the similarity metric of Sect. 1.4.1.

1.4.3 Clustering: Fuzzy C-Means (FCM)

FCM [9] is based on the minimization of an objective function defined as:

Table 1.2 Laplacian Eigenmap

Action	1	2	3
1	0.1690	0.1355	0.3829
2	0.1690	−0.0385	0.1308
3	0.1690	0.1667	−0.3825
4	0.1690	0.0625	0.1223
5	0.1690	0.1637	−0.0925

$$J_{FCM}(X; U, V) = \sum_{i=1}^{c} \sum_{j=1}^{N} \left(u_{ij}\right)^{m} D_{ij}$$

where N is the number of data points in the dataset, c is the pre-determined number of clusters, $X = [x_1, \cdots x_n]$ is the dataset matrix, $U = [u_{ij}]_{c*N}$ is the fuzzy membership matrix, $U_{ij} \in [0, 1]$ is the membership degree of the j-th data in the i-th cluster, $\sum_{i=1}^{c} u_{ij} = 1$, $V = [v_1, \cdots v_c]$, is the cluster prototype (centre) matrix, $m \in (1, \infty)$ is the weighting exponent (fuzzy index) which determines the fuzziness of the clusters and is usually set to 2, D_{ij} is the distance measure between data x_i and cluster prototype v_i. Typically, an $L2$ norm distance $D_{ijA} = ||x_j - v_i||_A^2 = (x_j - v_i)^T A(x_j - v_i)$ is used, where A is the norm-inducing matrix, usually taken to be the identity matrix.

Statistically, the objective function can be seen as a measure of the total variance of X_j from V_i. The minimization could be solved by using a variety of methods for nonlinear optimization problems.

The application to intention recognition produces clusters corresponding to the intentions in the plan library, one cluster for each intention. Figure 1.4 is based on the plan library of Table 1.1. It shows (fuzzy) clusters and their prototypes resulting from the application of FCM and Laplacian Eigenmap visualization using eigenvectors two and three of Table 1.2 (extended for all the actions). The bottom right (blue) cluster corresponds to intention 1, the top right (red) cluster corresponds to intention 2, and the left (yellow) cluster corresponds to intention 3. The cluster prototypes are denoted by hollow circles.

1.4.4 Intention Recognition and Membership Matrix

The iterative clustering algorithm, illustrated by fuzzy c-means above, provides not only the clusters, but also a membership matrix showing the probability of the membership of each action in each cluster. Table 1.3 shows the membership matrix based on the working example of Table 1.1 and the clusters in Fig. 1.4. The membership matrix is then used to accumulate scores for the intentions as actions are observed.

Given a sequence of actions, we simply sum up the membership values of these actions for each intention. The intentions with the highest scores are the most likely

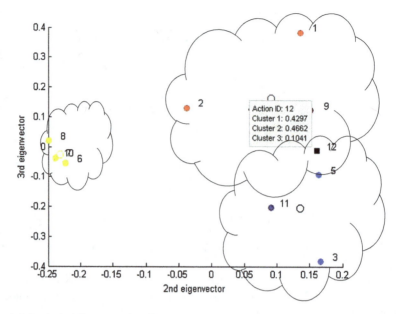

Fig. 1.4 Laplacian Eigenmap visualization using two eigenvectors

Table 1.3 Membership matrix

Action →	1	2	3	4	5	6	7	8	9	10	11	12
Intention ↓												
1	0.1135	0.0888	0.8185	0.0194	0.7797	0.0062	0.0012	0.0115	0.0446	0.0012	0.9710	0.4288
2	0.7563	0.7054	0.0887	0.9605	0.1545	0.0064	0.0014	0.0168	0.9273	0.0014	0.0147	0.4670
3	0.1302	0.2058	0.0928	0.0201	0.0657	0.9874	0.9974	0.9717	0.0281	0.9974	0.0143	0.1042

intentions. Figure 1.5 shows how the scores of the intentions changes as more actions are observed. The lines in the graph from top to bottom correspond to intentions 1, 2 and 3, respectively.

1.4.5 Other Clustering Algorithms

1.4.5.1 Possibilistic C-means (PCM)

A problem with FCM is that noise points usually lie far but equidistant from the cluster prototypes and are given equal membership values for all clusters. But such points should be given very low (even zero) value in each cluster. The Possibilistic C-Means [17] has been designed to overcome this problem. PCM relaxes the fuzzy membership matrix constraint $\sum_{i=1}^{c} u_{ij} = 1$ to obtain a "possibilistic" membership

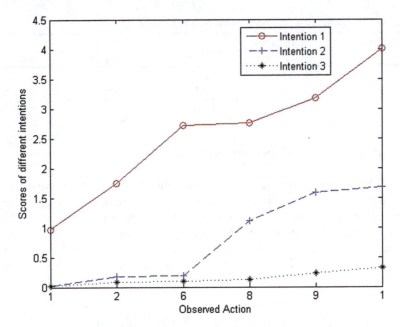

Fig. 1.5 Incremental intention recognition

constraint, $0 < \sum_{i=1}^{c} u_{ij} < c$. The objective function for PCM is defined as:

$$J_{PCM}(\mathbf{X}; \mathbf{U}, \mathbf{V}) = \sum_{i=1}^{c} \sum_{j=1}^{N} (u_{ij})^m D_{ij} + \sum_{i=1}^{c} \eta_i \sum_{j=1}^{N} (1 - u_{ij})^m,$$

where

$$\eta_i = K \frac{\sum_{j=1}^{N} (u_{ij})^m D_{ij}}{\sum_{j=1}^{N} (u_{ij})^m}, 1 \leq i \leq c$$

is the scale parameter at the i-th cluster. K is typically chosen to be 1. The first term of the objective function demands that the distances from data to the cluster prototype be as low as possible, whereas the second term forces the to be as large as possible to avoid trivial solutions. The value of determines when the membership value of a point in a cluster becomes 0.5.

Table 1.4 illustrates how PCM can give a different result compared to FCM, assuming a dataset with two noise points, A and B, and two clusters, where FCM would give values of 0.5 for the membership of each noise point in each cluster, and PCM can be more discriminating.

Table 1.4 Membership value of point A and B from FCM and PCM

Membership value	FCM		PCM	
	Cluster 1	Cluster 2	Cluster 1	Cluster 2
Point A	0.5	0.5	0.1363	0.1363
Point B	0.5	0.5	0.0586	0.0586

1.4.5.2 Improved Possibilistic C-means (IPCM)

Although PCM improves on FCM it can cause coincident clusters, i.e. two or more cluster prototypes can settle at the same position. In order to solve this problem Zhang and Leung [26] proposed an improved PCM algorithm which integrates FCM into the objective function. This combination can determine proper clusters as well as achieve robustness against noisy data. The improved PCM algorithm is derived directly from the possibilistic approach. The objective function of IPCM is defined as:

$$J_{IPCM}(\mathbf{X}; \mathbf{U}^{(P)}, \mathbf{U}^{(f)}, \mathbf{V}) = \sum_{i=1}^{c}\sum_{j=1}^{N}\left(u_{ij}^{(f)}\right)^{m_f}\left(\left(u_{ij}^{(p)}\right)^{m_p}D_{ij} + \eta_i\left(1 - u_{ij}^{(p)}\right)^{m_p}\right)$$

For further details we refer the reader to [26].

1.5 Empirical Results

1.5.1 Test Data

Two inputs are required for the intention recognition algorithm, namely the plan library and a sequence of observed actions to be classified. Regarding the plan library, many parameters can be varied. We vary two, *plan diversification (PD)*, that is how similar the plans for each intention are to each other, and *intention relatedness (InR)*, that is how similar the plans for an intention are to plans for other intentions. PD ranges from 0 to 1, such that for example, if it is 0.1 and the plan size is 100, then any two plans aiming for the same intention differ in 10 actions. For InR, the plans for different intentions consist of actions randomly chosen from an action set according to the Gaussian distribution $\mathcal{N}(\mu, \sigma^2)$. For example, if the actions set has 100 actions and the three Gaussian distributions are $\mathcal{N}(25, 5)$, $\mathcal{N}(50, 5)$, $\mathcal{N}(75, 5)$, the generated plans may have most of the actions around action 25, 50 and 75. The variance σ^2 determines the relatedness between different intentions.

Regarding the observed actions again several parameters can be varied. We vary two, the degrees of noise and partiality. We vary the noise parameter from 0 to 1, where 0 means there is no noise in the observed actions, while 1 means the whole sequence is randomly generated. Similarly, we vary the partiality parameter from 0 to 1, corresponding to the ratio of missing actions in the sequence.

We use an action set with 500 different actions, three intentions, each with three plans, and each plan having 150 actions. For intention relatedness we use three Gaussian distributions $\mathcal{N}(125, 75)$, $\mathcal{N}(250, 75)$, $\mathcal{N}(375, 75)$. For each intention, its plans are formed from actions randomly picked from the action set according to the distribution of the intention.

1.5.2 Experiments

1.5.2.1 Effectiveness of all Three Clustering Algorithms

We use nine sequences of observed actions, OA1-OA9, such that OA1-OA3 are predominantly related to intention 1 (I1), according to different plans of I1, OA4-OA6 to intention 2 (I2) and OA7-OA9 to intention 3 (I3). Table 1.5 shows the result for the most basic case where OA1-OA9 are non-noisy and non-partial. The plan diversification is 0.5. The figures in the table show the likelihood of each intention given the observation (likelihoods multiplied by 10 for easier readability). As shown the results are good. Similar results are obtained with noisy and partial observations for all three algorithms for all plan diversifications we tried (0.2, 0.5, 0.8). Some of these additional results are further illustrated in the next section.

1.5.2.2 Comparison of the Three Clustering Algorithms

To see how performances vary according to the degrees of noise, partialness and plan diversification we define a score r as the ratio of the score of the dominant intention (the one the algorithm assigns the highest value to) to the sum of the scores of all the intentions:

$$r = \frac{Score_{domIntention}}{\sum_{|I|} Score}$$

Figure 1.6 shows the relative performance of the three clustering algorithms under varying plan diversification, degrees of noise and degrees of partialness of observations. The bars with vertical stripes correspond to FCM, the bars with horizontal bars correspond to PCM, and the bars with diagonal lines correspond to IPCM.

From Fig. 1.6 we can see that overall IPCM has the best performance in all cases. With the increase of the diversification, generally the accuracy of PCM decreases. We believe this is because in diversified plans the cluster prototypes tend to move together in PCM.

With increasing degrees of noise the performance of all the algorithms declines somewhat, as one may expect. For a less diversified plan library, PCM performs

Table 1.5 Performance of the three clustering algorithms with non-noisy and non-partial observations, with plan diversification 0.5

		OA1	OA2	OA3	OA4	OA5	OA6	OA7	OA8	OA9
FCM	I1	118.34	102.93	105.34	18.75	21.48	22.66	12.30	24.50	19.55
	I2	18.68	26.78	22.06	110.24	105.06	98.41	19.55	17.26	24.65
	I3	12.98	20.29	22.60	21.01	23.46	28.93	118.14	108.24	105.80
Likeliest		I1	I1	I1	I2	I2	I2	I3	I3	I3
PCM	I1	96.12	86.72	89.57	18.94	20.40	3.45	15.78	24.02	20.52
	I2	20.53	25.50	23.44	87.88	82.09	96.64	21.19	19.60	24.39
	I3	16.91	21.22	24.02	20.56	22.29	49.91	96.39	88.85	89.33
Likeliest		I1	I1	I1	I2	I2	I2	I3	I3	I3
IPCM	I1	42.44	44.31	42.69	3.18	3.63	4.30	2.35	5.24	4.00
	I2	4.88	6.63	6.25	44.72	39.22	45.71	4.97	4.39	6.21
	I3	4.01	5.74	7.89	5.38	6.55	8.77	52.83	47.91	51.73
Likeliest		I1	I1	I1	I2	I2	I2	I3	I3	I3

Table 1.6 Summary of different clustering algorithms for intention recognition

Algorithm	Advantage	Disadvantage
FCM	Robust in noise-free environment	Sensitive to noise; Sensitive to initialization[a]
PCM	Able to cluster noisy data samples	Coincident cluster prototypes may occur; Sensitive to initialization
IPCM	Robust to noisy and partial observations	Sensitive to initialization

[a] Sensitive to initialization means that given random initialization of the cluster prototypes, the algorithm may easily get into local optima. It is better to initialize the algorithm based on any pre-knowledge of the positions of the prototypes

slightly better than FCM. All three algorithms perform better in the presence of partial observations than in the presence of noise. We conjecture that this is due to the fact that, depending on the levels of plan diversification and intention relatedness, even with partial observations we have a chance of seeing "typical" actions, which accumulatively help the algorithms to guess the correct intention.

Table 1.6, summarises our conclusions.

1.6 Conclusion and Future Work

We have explored the application of clustering techniques to the task of intention recognition, and have found the approach promising. We have also explored the suitability of three clustering algorithms, and found one, IPCM, the best fit for the task.

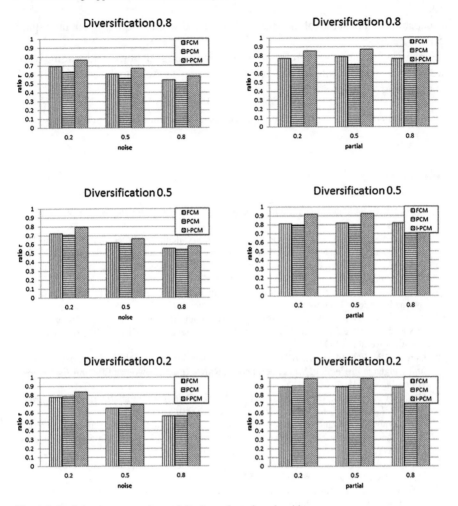

Fig. 1.6 Performance comparison of the three clustering algorithms

There is much more that can be explored in bridging the two fields of clustering and intention recognition. Other ways of computing similarity between actions can be investigated. There are several possibilities, for example assigning similarity in terms of resources the actions use, or the locations of actions, or their semantics via an action or causal theory, such as the event calculus [16].

Furthermore, the work reported in this chapter does not take into account the order of observed actions. However, such ordering information is useful in recognizing intentions. We have done some preliminary work in post-processing the results obtained from clustering to modify the likelihood of intentions according to the order of observed actions and other contextual constraints, such as the time of day, the capabilities and habits of the observed agent and so on. There is much more that needs to be done.

Finally, and crucially, more systematic testing for scalability, and testing with more realistic and meaningful data sets are necessary to evaluate the applicability of the clustering techniques further.

Acknowledgments We are grateful to the anonymous reviewers for their helpful comments.

References

1. Aarts, E., Ambient intelligence: a multimedia perspective. *IEEE Intelligent Systems 19(1)*, 12 19 (2004).
2. Baier, J. A., On procedure recognition in the Situation Calculus. In Proceedings of the Twelfth International Conference of the Chilean Computer Science Society (SCCC-02), 33–42 (2002).
3. Belkin, M. and Niyogi, P., Laplacian Eigenmapsfor Dimensionality Reductionand Data Representation, *Neural Computation* 15, 1373–1396 (2002).
4. Bui, H. H., A general model for online probabilistic plan recognition. In Proceedings of the International Joint Conference on, Artificial Intelligence (2003).
5. Cheng, D. C., Thawonmas, R., Case-based plan recognition for real-time strategy games. In Proceedings of the 5th Game-On International Conference (CGAIDE) 2004, Reading, UK, 36–40, November (2004).
6. Cohen, P.R., Perrault, C.R., Allen, J.F., Beyond question answering. In Strategies for Natural Language Processing, W. Lehnert and M. Ringle (Eds.), Lawrence Erlbaum Associates, Hillsdale, NJ, 245–274 (1981).
7. Cox, M.T., Kerkez, B., Case-Based Plan Recognition with Novel Input. International *Journal of Control and Intelligent Systems* 34(2), 96–104 (2006).
8. Demolombe, R., Fernandez, A.M.O., Intention recognition in the Situation Calculus and probability theory frameworks. In Proceedings of Computational Logic in Multi-agent Systems (CLIMA) (2006).
9. Dunn, J., A fuzzy relative of the ISODATA process and its use in detecting compact well separated clusters, *J. Cybern.* 3(3), 32–57 (1974).
10. Geib, C. W., Goldman, R. P., Plan recognition in intrusion detection systems. In the Proceedings of the DARPA Information Survivability Conference and Exposition (DISCEX), June (2001).
11. Geib, C. W., Goldman, R. P., Partial observability and probabilistic plan/goal recognition. In Proceedings of the International Workshop on Modeling Others from Observations (MOO-2005), July (2005).
12. Geib, C. W., Steedman, M., On natural language processing and plan recognition. In Proceedings of the International Joint Conference on Artificial Intelligence (IJCAI), 1612–1617 (2003).
13. Hong, J., Goal recognition through goal graph analysis, *Journal of Artificial Intelligence Research* 15, 1–30 (2001).
14. Jarvis, P., Lunt, T., Myers, K., Identifying terrorist activity with AI plan recognition technology. In the Sixteenth Innovative Applications of Artificial Intelligence Conference (IAAI 04), AAAI Press (2004).
15. Jolliffe, I. T., Principal Component Analysis. Springer, second ed., October (2002).
16. Kowalski, R. and Sergot, M., A Logic-based Calculus of Events, *New Generation Computing*, 4(1), 67–95 (1986).
17. Krishnapuram, R. and Keller, J., The possibilistic C-means algorithm: Insights and recommendations, *IEEE Transactions on Fuzzy Systems* 4, 385–393 (1996).

18. Levesque, H., Reiter, R., Lesperance, Y., Lin, F., Scherl, R., GOLOG: A Logic Programming Language for Dynamic Domains. *Journal of Logic Programming* 31, 59–84 (1997).
19. Mao, W., Gratch, J., A utility-based approach to intention recognition. AAMAS Workshop on Agent Tracking: Modelling Other Agents from Observations (2004).
20. Pereira, L.M., Anh, H.T., Elder care via intention recognition and evolution prospection, in: S. Abreu, D. Seipel (eds.), Procs. 18th International Conference on Applications of Declarative Programming and Knowledge Management (INAP'09), Évora, Portugal, November (2009).
21. Roy, P., Bouchard B., Bouzouane A, Giroux S., A hybrid plan recognition model for Alzheimer's patients: interleaved-erroneous dilemma. IEEE/WIC/ACM International Conference on Intelligent Agent Technology, 131–137 (2007).
22. Sadri, F., Logic-based Approaches to Intention Recognition, In Handbook of Research on Ambient Intelligence: Trends and Perspectives, Nak-Young Chong and Fulvio Mastrogiovanni Eds., IGI Global, May 2011, 346–375 (2011).
23. Sadri, F., Intention Recognition with Event Calculus Graphs and Weight of Evidence, Proc. of the 3rd International Conference on Agents and Artificial Intelligence, ed. J. Filipe, Springer January (2011).
24. Sadri, F., Intention Recognition in Agents for Ambient Intelligence: Logic-Based Approaches, to appear, Agent-Based Approaches to Ambient Intelligence, Bosse (ed.), IOS Press (2012).
25. Tenenbaum, J. B., de Silva, V. and Langford, J. C., A global geometric framework for nonlinear dimensionality reduction., *Science* 290, 2319–2323, December (2000).
26. Zhang, J. and Leung, Y., Improved possibilistic C-means clustering algorithms, IEEE *Transactions on Fuzzy Systems* 12(2), 209–217, April (2004).

Chapter 2
Adaptive Autonomy in Unmanned Ground Vehicles Using Trust Models

Armon Toubman, Peter-Paul van Maanen and Mark Hoogendoorn

Although autonomous systems are becoming more and more capable of performing tasks as good as humans can, there is still a huge amount of (especially) complex tasks which can much better be performed by humans. However, when making such task allocation decisions, it might show that in particular situations it is better to let a human perform the task, whereas in other situations an autonomous system might perform better. This could for instance depend upon the current state of the human, which might be measured by means of ambient devices, but also on experiences obtained in the past. In this chapter, a trust-based approach is developed which aims at judging the current situation and deciding upon the best allocation (to the human or autonomous system) of a certain task. Hereby, an experiment in the context of controlling a set of robots to dismantle bombs has been performed, with focus on multiple types of support. The results show that support by means of simply allocating the task to the most suitable party gives superior performance.

2.1 Introduction

Nowadays, more and more complex tasks that were originally performed by humans are being automated. This automation has become possible due to the huge advancements in technological development. For instance, in the field of robotics a trend can

A. Toubman (✉) · P.-P. van Maanen
Department of Cognitive Systems Engineering, TNO Human Factors, P.O. Box 23,
3769ZG Soesterberg, The Netherlands
e-mail: armon@armontoubman.com

P.-P. van Maanen · A. Toubman · M. Hoogendoorn
Department of Artificial Intelligence, Vrije Universiteit Amsterdam, De Boelelaan 1081a,
1081HV Amsterdam, The Netherlands
e-mail: peter-paul.vanmaanen@tno.nl

M. Hoogendoorn
e-mail: m.hoogendoorn@vu.nl

T. Bosse et al. (eds.), *Human Aspects in Ambient Intelligence*,
Atlantis Ambient and Pervasive Intelligence 8, DOI: 10.2991/978-94-6239-018-8_2,
© Atlantis Press and the authors 2013

be seen that moves from robots that were completely controlled by a human to robots that handle complete tasks autonomously [1]. Although the choice for automation might sometimes be clear-cut (e.g. robots mounting windows on cars are far more precise than humans) in other cases it might not be so obvious. For instance, it could be the case that an automated system performs far superiorly in straightforward situations, but in more complex situations a human might still perform better. Therefore, different so-called levels of autonomy (LOAs) can be defined ranging from complete control by the human to complete control by the autonomous system [2].

Currently, systems have been developed that try to accomplish an adaptive level of autonomy [3]. Such a system can take the form of an advice system for a human operator, but can also be an autonomous system itself that selects one of the LOAs. A key consideration when selecting one of these LOAs is the expected performance in a particular situation, both of the human and the automated system. In order to create these expectations, a performance model should be built up. Such a model should take previous experiences in similar situations into account, but can for instance also incorporate a model of the current state of the human operator (e.g. is the operator currently overloaded, or is the operator bored because he or she has nothing to do). In order to feed such a model with information, techniques from the domain of Ambient Intelligence can be deployed.

In this chapter, a first step in this direction is made in the field of robot control, by utilizing a computational trust model [4] to create a support system for a human operator. This system maintains a trust model for both the human operator and the automated system and derives which is better equipped to handle the current task. These trust levels are based on a history of experiences. The setting that is investigated does not concern a single but multiple robots that need to be controlled simultaneously, creating a situation where the human operator has to rely on the autonomous functions of the robots. The role of the human is shifted from operator to supervisor. In an experiment different forms of support are provided, ranging from displaying the robots, providing advice on who should take control of a particular robot, to completely autonomous assignment of control. Of course, the fact that the supervisor cannot control more than one robot at the same time is taken into account.

This chapter is organized as follows. In Sect. 2.2, the proposed support model is described. The hypotheses about the application of the support model are listed in Sect. 2.3, and the method used to test these hypotheses is described in Sect. 2.4. The results are given in Sect. 2.5. The chapter is concluded with a discussion in Sect. 2.6.

2.2 Support Model

A support model is proposed that can be used to aid a supervisor with the supervision and control of multiple robots. The support model consists of two main parts: a set of trust models and an autonomy reasoner. With these parts, the support model is able to offer different types of support. The support model is used in the context of supervisor S monitoring $n > 1$ robots $R_1, \ldots, R_n$. For each robot R_n, the support model has two trust models: one trust model T_{R_n} to predict robot R_n's performance, and one trust model T_{S_n} to predict the supervisor's performance when they are controlling robot R_n. The autonomy reasoner uses the trust values from the trust models to decide which robots are allowed to function autonomously, and which robot's control should be shifted to the supervisor, if any. A graphical overview of the support model is given in Fig. 2.1a.

2.2.1 Trust Models

The support model uses multiple instantiations of the same trust model to calculate the trust it has in the supervisor and the robots (together: agents) regarding a certain task. The trust model calculates the trust $T_j(s, t)$ that the support model has in trustee $j \in \{S, R_1, \ldots, R_n\}$ at time step t, with $T_j(s, t)$ ranging between 0 and 1. The calculated trust $T_j(s, t)$ represents a prediction of an agent's performance on the task.

With n robots, the support model uses $2n$ instantiations of the trust model. The performance of a robot R_n is predicted using a trust model T_{R_n}. Similarly, the performance of the supervisor when controlling each robot is predicted using trust models T_{S_n}.

The trust models use direct experiences and situations as input.

2.2.1.1 Direct Experiences

At every time step t, each trust model receives input in the form of either a positive or a negative experience, or no experience at all. Experiences are modeled in the support model as entities without explicit value. To discriminate between positive and negative experiences, each trust model remembers positive and negative experiences by maintaining two sets (Pos and Neg). From these sets, two new sets ($PosR$ and $NegR$) which contain only recent experiences are deduced at each time step:

$$
\begin{aligned}
Pos &= \{x | x \text{ is a time step at which a positive experience was received}\} \\
Neg &= \{x | x \text{ is a time step at which a negative experience was received}\} \\
PosR &= \{x \in Pos : x > t - \theta_t\} \\
NegR &= \{x \in Neg : x > t - \theta_t\}
\end{aligned}
\tag{2.1}
$$

The parameter θ_t defines after how many time steps an experience is no longer counted as recent. To let experiences with an agent influence the trust in that agent, the value of recent experiences needs to be quantified. This is done by looking at the ratio of positive experiences to negative experiences at each time step:

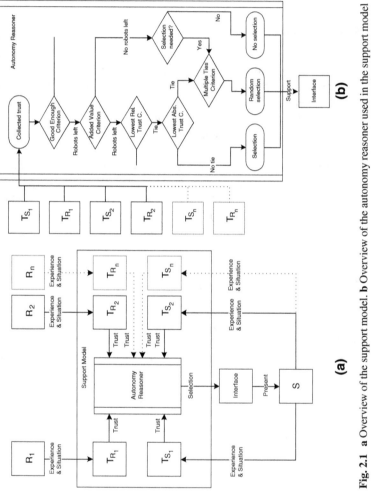

Fig. 2.1 **a** Overview of the support model. **b** Overview of the autonomy reasoner used in the support model

$$\varepsilon_j(t) = \begin{cases} \dfrac{\#PosR}{\#PosR + \omega_{neg}\#NegR} & \text{if } \#PosR + \#NegR > 0 \\ 0.5 & \text{otherwise} \end{cases} \qquad (2.2)$$

Here, ω_{neg} is a weight that can be used to balance the importance of negative experiences.

2.2.1.2 Situation

Combinations of features of the robots' environment, together with known properties of the robots, can form cues for the robots' expected performance. Such features make up situations. For example, a robot designed for urban warfare may have trouble moving through a desert area. It might be that this robot's wheels cannot drive through sand, or that its sensors cannot operate in high temperatures. Therefore, at each moment, performance predictions can be made with only knowledge of the robot's properties and its environment. In the trust models, scores are assigned to situations so that situations with a positive outlook add trust, while situations with a negative outlook subtract trust. The specific situations and their scores are defined before any operation as possible combinations of features of j's environment. The defined situations are assigned scores that indicate the outlook offered by the different situations, ranging from negative (a score of 0) to positive (a score of 1). The trust model for j obtains the score of j's situation with a lookup function:

$$\sigma_j(s, t) = \begin{cases} \text{The score of } s \text{ at } t \text{ if } s \text{ is a defined situation} \\ 0.5 \qquad\qquad\qquad\qquad \text{otherwise} \end{cases} \qquad (2.3)$$

The t parameter is used to reflect the declining or increasing predictive value of a situation as time passes. For example, if a robot spends too much time in a situation with a positive outlook (compared to the expected task completion time), trust in the robot declines as the amount of time spent might indicate a failure.

2.2.1.3 Combination of the Input

Direct experiences with j and j's situation at time step t have to be combined to form the new input I on which the trust in j at time step t is based:

$$I_j(s, t) = \omega_I \sigma_j(s, t) + (1 - \omega_I)\varepsilon_j(t) \qquad (2.4)$$

To be able to balance the importance of the experiences and the situation in the model, weight ω_I is introduced ($0 \le \omega_I \le 1$).

2.2.1.4 Final Definition

The final definition of the trust model is as follows:

$$T_j(s, t) = \lambda_T T_j(t - 1) + (1 - \lambda_T) I_j(s, t) \tag{2.5}$$

A decay factor λ_T ($0 \leq \lambda_T \leq 1$) is added to control how strongly old trust influences new trust.

With $2n$ instantiations of this trust model, the support model is able to predict the performance of each robot, and the performance of the supervisor with each robot. These predictions, in the form of trust values, form the input of the autonomy reasoner, which is described in the next section.

2.2.2 Autonomy Reasoner

The autonomy reasoner uses the trust values generated by the trust models to select (at most) one robot at each time step. The selected robot is the most suitable candidate for a shift in control, according to the support model. A number of criteria are applied on the trust values that enter the autonomy reasoner.

First, threshold θ_1 ($0 < \theta_1 < 1$) is defined as the trust value for each T_{R_i} above which robot R_i should not be considered further for a control shift. This can be formalized as the first criterion for the autonomy reasoner:

Criterion 1.1 (Good Enough). *For each robot R_i, if $T_{R_i} > \theta_1$, remove R_i from consideration for selection.*

While the predicted performance of a robot may be low ($\leq \theta_1$), the difference with the predicted performance of the supervisor with that robot might not be large enough to warrant a shift in control. A new threshold θ_2 ($0 < \theta_2 < \theta_1 < 1$) is needed for the maximum difference in trust in the robot and the supervisor under which R_i is allowed to retain control, when $T_{R_i} \leq \theta_1$. The second criterion can now be defined:

Criterion 1.2 (Added Value). *For each robot R_i, if $T_{S_i} - T_{R_i} < \theta_2$, remove R_i from consideration for selection.*

From the robots that are still being considered, the autonomy reasoner selects the robot that is expected to perform the worst relative to the supervisor:

Criterion 1.3 (Lowest Relative Trust). *Find the distinct $\arg\max_i (T_{S_i} - T_{R_i})$ and select robot R_i.*

It is possible that multiple robots are tied for the lowest relative trust, meaning the Lowest Relative Trust Criterion can not select a single robot. In this case, the robot in which the support model has the lowest absolute trust should be selected:

Criterion 1.4 (Lowest Absolute Trust). *Find the distinct* $\arg\min_i (T_{R_i})$ *and select robot* R_i.

Again a tie is possible. In case of a tie with the Lowest Absolute Trust Criterion, a random robot is selected:

Criterion 1.5 (Multiple Ties). *Robot* R_i *is selected at random, and this selection is maintained until the next time step at which a robot is selected by application of any criterion except the Multiple Ties Criterion.*

If after application of the Added Value Criterion no robots are left for consideration for selection, a shift in control is not deemed necessary by the autonomy reasoner. However, if a shift is required, a selection can be forced by applying the Multiple Ties Criterion on all robots.

A graphical overview of the autonomy reasoner is given in Fig. 2.1b.

2.2.3 Support Types

Three types of support using the support model are proposed: Trust Overview, Weak Adaptive Autonomy and Strong Adaptive Autonomy.

As the first type of support (Trust Overview), the trust generated by T_{R_i} for each robot i can be presented to the supervisor. The autonomy reasoner is bypassed. The supervisor must make all decisions about the robots' autonomy themselves. The presentation of the trust values can be used as a decision aid.

As the second type of support (Weak Adaptive Autonomy), the support model is used as shown in Fig. 2.1a. At each time step t, the trust in all agents is updated and a selection is made by the autonomy reasoner. This selection is presented to the supervisor as the most suitable candidate for a shift of control to the supervisor.

As the third type of support (Strong Adaptive Autonomy), the support model is again used as shown in Fig. 2.1a. However, the selected robot is not merely presented to the supervisor. The supervisor is forced to take control of the selected robot. At each time step t, the trust in all agents is updated and a selection is made by the autonomy reasoner. The choice of whether to shift control of a robot to the supervisor is taken from the supervisor. Instead, the control of the selected robot is forced on the supervisor by the support model.

2.3 Hypotheses

Several hypotheses can be formed on the effectiveness of the support types offered by the support model that was described in the previous section.

The support model was designed to help the supervisor monitor robots and decide over their autonomy. The support model, using trust models, should be able to more accurately predict the performance of robots than the supervisor. Therefore, the supervisor/robot team is expected to achieve higher performance in their tasks when the supervisor is supported with either Trust Overview (H1a), Weak Adaptive Autonomy (H1b), or Strong Adaptive Autonomy (H1c), compared to when the supervisor does not receive support. Specifically, team performance is expected to be the highest when the supervisor is supported by Strong Adaptive Autonomy (H2). In other words, the support model should be able to make better decisions on the robots' autonomy than the supervisor.

The support model uses trust models to predict the performance of robots. Since trust is a subjective measure, the only baseline suitable for comparison is that of human opinion. The support model's predictions and decisions can be compared to human opinion in two ways.

First, the trust the support model has in the robots and the supervisor can be compared to the trust a human would have, when given the same information as the support model to base their trust on. The expectation of increased team performance can be reduced into the expectation that the trust models used by the support model are better at predicting performance than the method used by humans. Therefore, trust generated by the support model is not expected to resemble trust reported by humans (H3), given the same information as input.

Second, the decisions of the support model on the autonomy of the robots (in the form of the robots selected by the switching mechanism) can be compared to the decisions of the supervisors in the same situations. For higher team performance with support from the support model, supervisors need to agree with the advice from the support model. Meanwhile, supervisors' agreement is expected to be low without support from the support model—if it were high, there would be no added benefit in application of the support model. Therefore, it is hypothesized that supervisors will agree with the advice from the support model (under Trust Overview and Weak Adaptive Autonomy) (H4). When no support is given, supervisors are not expected to agree with the selected robot the support model would have provided.

2.4 Method

2.4.1 Participants

Thirty-five experienced computer users participated in the experiment ($M = 30.5$ years, $\sigma = 13.4$ years, 17 female). Out of each group of five participants, four were randomly assigned the role of supervisor.

2.4.2 Task

To test the hypotheses from Sect. 2.3, a task has been designed in which four robots have to disarm as many bombs as possible at a priori unknown locations at the same time in separate virtual mazes. These four robots were supervised by a human supervisor. The robots themselves were operated by humans (as opposed to an AI algorithm, which (1) would have required more effort to program, (2) does not represent future AI capabilities anyway, and (3) the focus of the experiment was on the supervisor's task, not the robot operators' task). The robot operators were not able to communicate with the supervisor. The supervisor monitored the activity of the robots and was able to shift the control of one robot at a time to himself.

To add realism to the task (i.e., a certain degree of uncertainty of properly finding and disarming bombs) there were three types of bombs in each maze: (1) bombs that only the robot operators could see, (2) bombs that only the supervisor could see and (3) bombs that both could see. In this way both parties (robot operator and supervisor) would have their own capabilities and needed each other to take over control at different moments in time to have an optimal performance.

A bomb was disarmed (positive experience) when a robot drove over it when visible to its current controller. When a robot drove over a bomb that was not visible to its current controller, the bomb exploded (negative experience). Both the operator and supervisor were notified whenever one of these events happened. A bomb visible on the interface constituted a positive situation. If no bomb was picked up after 20 s of seeing one, the situation became neutral, and after 20 more seconds, the situation became negative until a bomb was picked up.

Control of a robot was required in order to see bombs. Also a shift of control to the supervisor required 5 s to process. These two measures were needed to prevent the supervisor from micro-managing the robots too easily (i.e., quickly take over control, disarm a bomb and release control whenever a bomb is seen by the supervisor).

Each maze contained the same number of bombs. However, the number of bombs of each type differed per robot in each trial. This caused each robot to have a different performance, giving the supervisor reason to pay close attention to the performance of each robot. The less bombs visible to a robot, the more difficult that robot's task is: it will find less bombs to disarm and have a higher chance of causing explosions. The same holds for the supervisor. Four combinations of bombs were used: one with most bombs visible to the robot operator, one setup with most bombs visible to the supervisor, one setup with most bombs visible to both, and one setup with an equal division. An overview of the bomb setups that were used can be found in Table 2.1. The bomb combinations were balanced between the robots in the four rounds under each supervisor. The balancing scheme is shown in Table 2.2.

The interface for the robot operators is shown in Fig. 2.2a. It shows the robot's immediate surroundings. The operator was able to steer the robot through its maze using the WASD keys. Bombs were displayed as a red circle. When the robot drove over a visible bomb, a green indicator would appear for a short time, accompanied by a sound. When the robot drove over an invisible bomb, a red indicator would appear,

Table 2.1 Overview of the bomb combinations

Combination	Visible by robot operator	Visible by supervisor	Visible by both
1	+	−	−
2	−	+	−
3	−	−	+
4	☐	☐	☐

Table 2.2 Bomb combination Latin square

Trial number under same supervisor	Bomb combination for robot			
	1	2	3	4
1	1	2	3	4
2	2	4	1	3
3	3	1	4	2
4	4	3	2	1

(a)

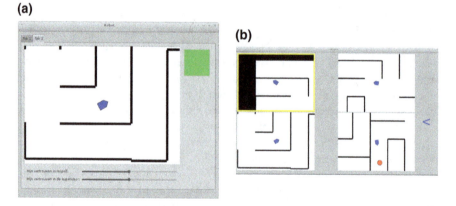

Fig. 2.2 **a** Robot operator's interface. **b** Supervisor's interface

accompanied by a different sound. When the robot was controlled by the supervisor, the same indicators and sounds were used for these events.

The interface contained a large colored indicator that showed who was in control of the robot: the robot operator or the supervisor. The indicator would switch between green (the operator controls the robot) and red (the supervisor controls the robot). Control switches were also accompanied by a clear sound.

The supervisor's interface let the supervisor monitor the activity of the robots and take control of one robot at a time. Support from the support model was also given through this interface. The different implementations of these types of support (as explained in Sect. 2.2.3 is further described in Sect. 2.4.3.1. The interface is shown in Fig. 2.2b.

Table 2.3 Experimental design

Supervisor	Conditions			
1	NS	TO	WAA	SAA
2	TO	SAA	NS	WAA
3	WAA	NS	SAA	TO
4	SAA	WAA	TO	NS

2.4.3 Design

A 4 × 1 within subjects design was used. The single independent variable used in the design was the type of support offered by the support model. This resulted in four conditions, named after the support types: NS (No Support), TO (Trust Overview), WAA (Weak Adaptive Autonomy), and SAA (Strong Adaptive Autonomy).

The order in which the conditions were presented to the supervisors were balanced with a Latin square, as shown in Table 2.3.

2.4.3.1 Independent Variables

The single independent variable that was manipulated in the experiment was the type of support offered by the support model as explained in Sect. 2.2.3. Figure. 2.2b shows the 'Weak Adaptive Autonomy' condition, which shows all components used in all conditions. Details specific to each support type are given below.

No Support: Under this setting, the supervisor received no support from the support model. The supervisor had to measure each robot's performance manually by paying attention to the red and green indicators that accompanied disarmaments and explosions. The supervisor was able to take and give back control of robots at will.

Trust Overview: Under this setting, the level of trust the trust models of the support model had in each robot was presented to the supervisor as a colored border around the window with each robot's activity. The color of each border represented the level of trust the support model had in that robot. The borders blended gradually between red (low trust), yellow (medium trust) and green (high trust). The supervisor was able to take and give back control of robots at will. The supervisor was instructed to consider the colored borders as performance predictors.

Weak Adaptive Autonomy: Under this setting, the support model selected a robot which should be taken over by the supervisor, and presented the selection to the supervisor.

The indicator for the chosen robot was a colored border around the window with the chosen robot's activity. The color of the border represented the level of trust the support model had in that robot. The border blended gradually between red (low trust), yellow (medium trust) and green (high trust). The supervisor was instructed to consider the robot that was selected by the support model. as the support model expected this robot to increase team performance the most with a control shift.

The autonomy reasoner in the support model was configured to always select a robot. This was done to keep supervisors involved in the operation. The trials were short, creating the possibility that the supervisor would not receive advice during a whole trial. Because the autonomy reasoner always had to select a robot, it was chosen to include the trust in the selected robot in the presentation of the selection (see Sect. 2.2.3).

Strong Adaptive Autonomy: Under this setting, the support model selected a robot which should be taken over by the supervisor. The supervisor was forced to comply with this decision. The selected robot was indicated with a blue arrow.

2.4.3.2 Dependent Variables

Team performance: Three measures were used to calculate the performance of the supervisor-robots team on the task.

The first measure was the number of bombs that was disarmed (hits). The number of disarmed bombs should be maximized. The higher the amount of bombs disarmed by the team, the higher the team's performance was.

The second measure was the number of bombs that was set off (misses). The number of bombs set off should be minimized. The lower the amount of bombs set off by the team, the higher the team's performance was.

The third measure combined the previous two measures. The z-scores of both the number of bombs disarmed and the number of bombs set off were calculated per condition. The z-score of the number of bombs set off was then subtracted from the number of bombs disarmed, resulting in a normalized measure of performance per condition. The third measure can be seen as a more objective measure than the first and second measures. Averaging the performance values of all trials per condition resulted in mean performance values for each condition.

Similarity of trust: Trust was obtained in two forms: trust generated by the trust models and trust estimates from the robot operators.

Each trial, the trust models in the support model generated eight sets of trust values: trust in each of the four robot operators and four times trust in the supervisor.

Also during each trial, robot operators had to indicate their trust in themselves and in their supervisor using on-screen slider controls (as shown at the bottom of Fig. 2.2a). The slider controls had eleven-point scales. The participants were reminded every thirty seconds with spoken text to update the sliders if they felt their trust had changed. This resulted in eight pairs of trust datasets from each trial. The root mean square deviation (RMSD) was calculated for the pairs of these datasets with the same trustee (the robot operator or the supervisor). This yielded two sets of RMSDs, one set for each trustee.

Agreement: This shows how often the supervisor agreed with the support model by looking at which robots the supervisor took control of and what the support model had advised to take over (depending on the type of support).

Condition	μ	σ	$\mu > \mu_{NS}$		
			t	df	Sig.
NS	56.6111	7.9049	–	–	–
TO	55.8333	8.4523	−0.5416	17	0.7024
WAA	57.2778	6.4790	0.3816	17	0.3537
SAA	60.6667	9.2036	2.2886	17	0.0176

Table 2.4 Statistical reports on team performance as the number of disarmed bombs per condition

2.5 Results

2.5.1 Removal of Outliers

Out of the data from 28 supervisors, the data from 10 supervisors was removed because the number of disarmed or exploded bombs was higher or lower than two standard deviations from the mean performance.

2.5.2 Team Performance

Team performance was calculated using three measures: the number of disarmed bombs (hits), the number of exploded bombs (misses), and a normalized score.

The first measure was the number of disarmed bombs. Details of the four conditions are given in Table 2.4. The mean number of disarmed bombs per condition is shown in Fig. 2.3a. A repeated measures ANOVA showed no significant effect of condition on performance, $F(3, 51) = 2.5$, $p = 0.0695$. Paired sample t-tests indicated a significantly higher performance under SAA compared to NS. This was not the case with TO and WAA. The highest mean number of disarmed bombs was achieved under SAA.

The second measure was the number of exploded bombs. Details of the four conditions are given in Table 2.5. The mean number of exploded bombs per condition is shown in Fig. 2.3b. A repeated measures ANOVA showed a significant effect of condition on performance, $F(3, 51) = 4.27$, $p = 0.0092$. Paired sample t-tests indicated no significantly higher performance under any of the conditions with support from the support model. The lowest mean number of exploded bombs was achieved under SAA.

The third measure was the normalized score. Details of the four conditions are given in Table 2.6. The mean number of exploded bombs per condition is shown in Fig. 2.3c. A repeated measures ANOVA showed a significant effect of condition on performance, $F(3, 51) = 5.12$, $p = 0.0036$. Paired sample t-tests indicated a significantly higher performance under SAA compared to NS. This was not the case with TO and WAA. The highest mean normalized score was achieved under SAA.

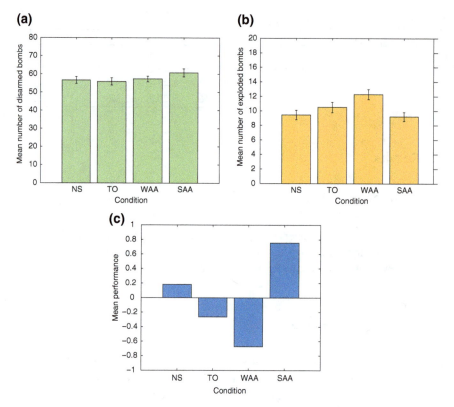

Fig. 2.3 **a** Mean number of disarmed bombs per condition. **b** Mean number of exploded bombs per condition. **c** Mean normalized team scores per condition

Table 2.5 Statistical reports on team performance as the number of exploded bombs per condition

Condition	μ	σ	$\mu < \mu_{NS}$		
			t	df	Sig.
NS	9.4444	2.7912	–	–	–
TO	10.5000	2.9754	1.1703	17	0.8710
WAA	12.2778	2.9267	2.5543	17	0.9897
SAA	9.2222	2.6022	−0.2827	17	0.3904

    The number of hits under SAA was significantly higher than the number of hits under No Support (NS), while the application of Trust Overview (TO) and Weak Adaptive Autonomy (WAA) did not significantly improve performance. Based on the results, hypotheses H1a and H1b are rejected, while hypothesis H1c is accepted. Furthermore, using each of the three performance measures, the highest performance was achieved under Strong Adaptive Autonomy (SAA). For this reason, hypothesis H2 is accepted.

Condition	μ	σ	$\mu > \mu_{NS}$		
			t	df	Sig.
NS	0.1818	1.2929	–	–	–
TO	−0.2633	1.4930	−1.5267	17	0.9274
WAA	−0.6735	1.3227	−2.0131	17	0.9699
SAA	0.7551	1.5399	2.0781	17	0.0266

Table 2.6 Statistical reports on team performance as normalized scores per condition

The increased performance under SAA shows that the support model can make better decisions on autonomy than human supervisors. This is supported by the performance under TO and WAA. The high performance under SAA shows that the advice given by the support model under TO and WAA was useful for basing decisions on.

2.5.3 Similarity of Trust

As described in Sect. 2.4.3.2, two times eight sets of trust values were collected each trial.

Two one-sample t-tests were conducted, comparing each set of RMSDs to a mean of 0. There was a significant difference for both the trust in the robot ($p = 0$, $a = 0.05$) and the trust in the supervisor ($p = 0$, $a = 0.05$).

Neither the trust of the supervisor and the trust models in the supervisor nor the trust in the robot operators correlated between the trustors. Therefore, hypothesis H3 is accepted.

2.5.4 Agreement

Each trial yielded two sets of data on the control of the robots: one set showing which robots the support model had selected, and one set showing which robots the supervisor actually took control of.

The agreement between the supervisor and the support model was calculated as Cohen's kappa for each trial except trials under Strong Adaptive Autonomy. This resulted in mean kappas for No Support ($\mu_\kappa = 0.0622$, $\sigma_\kappa = 0.1371$), Trust Overview ($\mu_\kappa = 0.1055$, $\sigma_\kappa = 0.1126$), and Weak Adaptive Autonomy ($\mu_\kappa = 0.1216$, $\sigma_\kappa = 0.1424$).

The agreement of the supervisor with the support model under NS, TO and WAA was low by any standard. Therefore, hypothesis H4 is rejected. Apparently, the method used by the supervisors to make decisions on the robots' autonomy was very different from the method used by the support model. A high agreement of the supervisors with the support model would show that the support model used a method comparable to the method used by the supervisors. However, this is clearly not the case.

2.6 Discussion

The main goal of this study was to find out if support from a support model that uses trust models would increase team performance in the case of a human supervisor monitoring multiple robots. Trust models have previously been used to provide support in different settings, but results have varied [5, 6]. In this study, a clear positive effect was found.

The most interesting result is that team performance was the highest under SAA. Apparently, the support model made better decisions on the LOAs of the robots than the human supervisors did. This result is coherent with the low agreement that was found between the supervisors and the support model, and also with the low correlation in trust.

One explanation for the higher performance under SAA is computational power. While the support model can monitor the robots and the supervisor without error, human supervisors have a limited attention capacity, meaning they may have missed or wrongly attributed events such as disarmaments of bombs, explosions, and changed situations. The wrong attribution of events could be explained with Weiner's attribution theory [7]. Supervisors may have attributed their own successes to skill, while attributing the robots' successes to luck. The support model made objective observations of the robots and the supervisors, leading to better decisions.

The low agreement of the supervisor with the support model's advice under the TO and WAA conditions can be regarded as under-reliance. Under-reliance remains a problem in the field of human-machine interaction [3]. Several factors could have contributed to the supervisors' under-reliance on the support model. Among these factors are an inadequate understanding of the method used by the support model to select robots, and the inability to access the raw information which the support model uses as input.

It should be noted that the configuration of the support model, which forced it to continuously select robots to prevent underload, may have influenced the supervisors' reliance on the advice under WAA. The selection of robots which were not in actual need of a control shift based on their predicted performance, may have been perceived by the supervisors as false alarms. In short, agreement under WAA may have been higher if the continuous selection of robots was disabled.

Some comments can be made on the inner workings of the support model. One such comment is about the used paradigm that positive experiences increase trust, and negative experiences decrease trust. This view is called naive and not useful for artificial systems, because it is unable to attribute successes and failures to their proper causes [8]. It is noted, however, that such a view cannot be avoided if the trust is modeled as a simple number. In the trust models used in the support model, trust was indeed modeled as a simple number. By using multiple trust models, the support model did avoid the naive view on attribution.

Another comment that can be made is that the values of the support model's parameters used in the implementation were chosen manually. Tuning the parameters may lead to even higher performance using the support model. Parameter tuning could be done offline before operation, but future research may also bring effective online parameter tuning techniques. This way, the support model and the support it provides could be made more adaptive to unknown and changing environments. The autonomy reasoner could also be made adaptive, for example with the exploration and exploitation method [9].

The proposed support model showed positive results when it was allowed to make all LOA decisions. The support in the form of advice can be improved. Future research should point out if the support model can be used effectively in different settings.

References

1. R. Parasuraman, T. B. Sheridan, C. D. Wickens, A Model for Types and Levels of Human Interaction with Automation, Systems, Man and Cybernetics, Part A: Systems and Humans, IEEE Transactions on. 30(3), (2000). doi:10.1109/3468.844354. URL http://dx.doi.org/10.1109/3468.844354
2. T. B. Sheridan and W. L. Verplank. Human and computer control of undersea teleoperators (Man-Machine Systems Laboratory Report), (1978).
3. R. Parasuraman and C. D. Wickens, Humans: Still Vital After All These Years of Automation, Human Factors: The Journal of the Human Factors and Ergonomics Society. 50(3), 511–520 (June, 2008). ISSN 0018–7208. doi:10.1518/001872008X312198. URL http://dx.doi.org/10.1518/001872008X312198
4. J. Sabater and C. Sierra, Review on Computational Trust and Reputation Models, Artif. Intell. Rev. 24, 33–60 (Sept., 2005). ISSN 0269–2821. URL http://portal.acm.org/citation.cfm?id=1057866
5. P.-P. van Maanen, T. Klos, and K. van Dongen, Aiding Human Reliance Decision Making Using Computational Models of Trust. pp. 372–376 (Nov., 2007). doi:10.1109/WI-IATW.2007.108. URL http://dx.doi.org/10.1109/WI-IATW.2007.108
6. P.-P. van Maanen, F. Wisse, J. van Diggelen, and R.-J. Beun. Effects of Reliance Support on Team Performance by Advising and Adaptive Autonomy. In Proceedings of the 2011 IEEE/WIC/ACM International Conference on Intelligent Agent Technology (IAT-2011). IEEE Computer Society Press, (2011).
7. B. Weiner, An Attributional Theory of Achievement Motivation and Emotion, Psychological Review. 92(4), 548–573 (Oct., 1985). ISSN 0033–295X. URL http://view.ncbi.nlm.nih.gov/pubmed/3903815
8. R. Falcone and C. Castelfranchi. Trust Dynamics: How Trust Is Influenced by Direct Experiences and by Trust Itself. In Proceedings of the Third International Joint Conference on Autonomous Agents and Multiagent Systems - Volume 2, AAMAS '04, pp. 740–747, Washington, DC, USA, (2004). IEEE Computer Society. ISBN 1-58113-864-4. doi:10.1109/AAMAS.2004.286. URL http://dx.doi.org/10.1109/AAMAS.2004.286
9. M. Hoogendoorn, S. W. Jaffry, J. Treur, Exploration and Exploitation in Adaptive Trust-Based Decision Making in Dynamic Environments, Web Intelligence and Intelligent Agent Technology, IEEE/WIC/ACM International Conference on. 2, 256–260, (2010). doi:10.1109/WI-IAT.2010.199. URL http://dx.doi.org/10.1109/WI-IAT.2010.199

Part II
Motion Tracking

Chapter 3
Automated Analysis of Non-Verbal Expressive Gesture

S. Piana, M. Mancini, A. Camurri, G. Varni and G. Volpe

3.1 Introduction

The work presented in this chapter is part of the EU FP7 ICT 3-year Project ASC-INCLUSION, that aims at developing ICT solutions to assist children affected by Autism Spectrum Conditions (ASC). In particular, it focuses on the development of serious games to support ASC-children in understanding and expressing emotions. The general ASC-INCLUSION framework will be able to process facial expressions, voice, and full-body movement and gesture. Automated monitoring of children behavior in ecological environments (e.g., home) is important to detect their emotional state and stimulate them to interact socially. The proposed system will monitor the ASC children while they are interacting with other people or playing serious games and will evaluate their ability to express and understand emotions. Then the system will try to help the children improve their knowledge of emotions using interactive multimodal feedback.

Previous work on the same topic include [1], in which authors evaluated an interactive software for teaching emotions to adults affected by autism and Asperger syndrome. The system has been then tested on children by [2, 3]. In [4, 5], emotions and facial expressions are taught through an animated series created to motivate

S. Piana (✉) · M. Mancini · A. Camurri · G. Varni · G. Volpe
Casa Paganini-InfoMus, University of Genoa, Genoa, Italy
e-mail: steto84@infomus.org

M. Mancini
e-mail: maurizio.mancini@dist.unige.it

A. Camurri
e-mail: antonio.camurri@unige.it

G. Varni
e-mail: giovannavarni@unige.it

G. Volpe
e-mail: gualtiero.volpe@unige.it

young children with ASC by embedding emotional content in a world populated by mechanical vehicles.

In the framework of the ASC-INCLUSION Project, in this chapter we focus on the system component and in particular on a general software architecture for non-verbal full-body automated behavior analysis. Section 3.2 presents state of the art on Kinect-based user tracking and analysis of movement. Section 3.3 presents a framework for performing users monitoring in multiple environments (e.g., rooms of a house), integrating the information on their behavior (e.g., to determine users' social roles) and finally provide an interactive audiovisual stimuli based on the users' behavior that is coherent with the ASC therapy.

Section 3.4 describes a software architecture corresponding to a subset of the presented framework based on the EyesWeb XMI platform, in which low, mid and high-level motion features from multiple users are extracted. Finally, Sect. 3.5 describes future work, aiming at understanding ASC children's emotional state and to create interactive systems to provide them an appropriate feedback.

3.2 Related Work

Several works explored the possible applications of the Kinect sensor human body tracking capabilities to research fields such as rehabilitation, social interaction and multimodal interfaces.

In two different works, Chang et al. [6, 7] assessed the possibility of, respectively, rehabilitating two young adults with motor impairments using a Kinect-based system in a public school setting and training individuals with cognitive impairments using a Kinect-based task prompting system. Raptis et al. [8] presented a real-time gesture classification system for skeletal wireframe motion. Albrektsen [9] conceived an innovative approach to social robotics through gesture recognition.

Authors of Leroy et al. [10] presented a system in which, by analyzing their behavior in realtime, the machine chooses which user to interact with. Users are tracked by a Kinect sensor and some social features are computed: the users' distance and velocity are compared to determine the most contrasted person in the group. The system's output, a big eye projected on a screen, is changed according to the most contrasted person (the big eye points to that person). In this way, authors aim to demonstrate that an intelligent machine could be capable of choosing within a small group of people the one it will interact with.

In Francese et al. [11] authors use the Kinect sensor to navigate onto 3D maps with body gestures by using the bird/airplane metaphor (arms stretched outside, raising/lowering/leaning arms) while in Cuccurullo et al. [12] authors show that PowerPoint presentation management could be improved by performing body gestures (e.g., raising/lowering one or two arms) and Kinect. In, [13] the Kinect interface tracks a single user's head and hands to determine user's body and hands' smoothness. Then a measure of entropy is computed on these motion features.

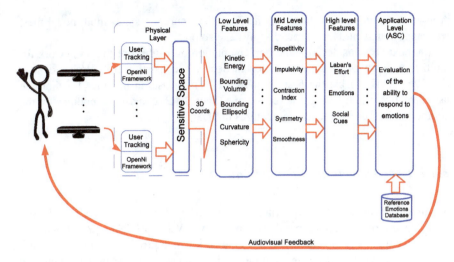

Fig. 3.1 Framework for multi-user non-verbal expressive gesture analysis

3.3 Multi-user Non-verbal Expressive Gesture Analysis Framework

This section describes a framework for multi-user non-verbal expressive gesture analysis; an overview of this framework is depicted in Fig. 3.1. The framework is based on a *multilayered conceptual framework* developed by Camurri and colleagues [14, 15]. Such framework supports multimodal systems, and includes a Physical Layer, in which data captured by sensors (e.g., images) is analyzed and early processing is performed. The choice of the Kinect sensor enables full-body (2D as well as 3D) user tracking. The support of multiple Kinect sensors, as shown in Fig. 3.1, allows one to track movement in a sensitive space wider than using a single Kinect sensor. That is, a higher number of users can be tracked simultaneously: each Kinect sensor focuses on a different space area, then the data captured by each device is merged to obtain a single sensitive area. The motion capture measurements provided by each Kinect are then managed and modified to share the same absolute reference system.

3.4 Software Architecture

The EyesWeb XMI platform is a modular system that allows both expert (e.g., researchers in computer engineering) and non-expert users (e.g., artists) to create multimodal installations in a visual way [19]. The platform provides modules, called *blocks*, that can be assembled intuitively (i.e., by operating only with mouse) to create programs, called *patches*, that exploit system's resources such as multimodal files, webcams, sound cards, multiple displays and so on.

The next sections describe the implementation of a subset of the framework for multi-user behavior analysis proposed in Sect. 3.3, consisting in 2 classes of new EyesWeb XMI blocks: the first one (Sect. 3.4.1) consists in modules for multiple user detection and tracking; the second one (Sect. 3.4.2) consists in modules for the computation of users' movement features in 3D.

3.4.1 User Detection and Tracking

Multiple users detection and tracking is performed by different EyesWeb XMI modules. The use of Kinect as input device in the EyesWeb XMI development platform is possible thanks to the OpenNI [20] framework which provides software modules for audio and video streaming from the device's sensors and for user tracking and user movement segmentation. Furthermore the EyesWeb XMI environment can:

- Support automated calibration of the user tracking system and provide functionalities to save configuration files. Such a feature allows one to avoid the tuning phase of the Kinect: the automated calibration phase requires a short period of time (10-15 s) where the tracking measurements are less precise; to avoid this process, the system can save and load calibration files to reduce the time needed for calibration.
- Save and load video recordings of the participants using ".oni" files. Such a format allows one to store both video data from the Kinect color camera and depth information from the Kinect depth sensor. The recorded streams can then be played and analyzed in order to extract user's tracking data (these functions are automatically done by software modules). The support for ONI files simplifies data recording for offline analysis.

The following EyesWeb XMI modules manage the communication between the EyesWeb XMI environment and the Kinect sensors and perform user's movement segmentation and tracking:

- KinectExtractor: provides input data from the Kinect sensor. Multiple instances of this block may be instantiated in the application in order to use several Kinect sensors at the same time. For each sensor, the output provided by the module consists of: the set of tracked users; the image from the color camera or, alternatively, the image from the infrared camera; an image representing the reconstructed depthmap, where the distance from the sensor is mapped to a gray-level in the image. The module KinectExtractor can, optionally, record all such data to an ONI file. It can be configured with the following parameters:

  (a) Kinect ID: identifies the Kinect device when multiple sensors are connected to the same system;

(b) Kinect tilt: controls the tilt angle of the Kinect sensor with respect to the horizontal plane;

(c) Image output: specifies whether the image from the color camera or from the infrared camera is provided as output;

(d) Image format: switches between the two currently supported image resolutions, i.e., 640×480 or 1024×768;

(e) Align depth map to image: since the color camera is slightly displaced with respect to the infrared camera (which is used to compute the depth map), the corresponding images might not be perfectly aligned. This parameter allows for compensation of this misalignment;

(f) Number of users: the maximum number of distinct users managed by the Kinect device;

(g) Skeleton type: specifies whether a body skeleton is computed by the block and its type (e.g., full body, upper half, etc.);

(h) Coordinates output type: specifies whether the coordinates of the skeleton computed by the block are in real word units (millimeters) or in image units (normalized in the range $0.0 - 1.0$);

(i) Confidence threshold: allow tuning of the reliability of the computed coordinates of the points of the skeleton. The points are added to the skeleton only if their measured level of confidence is beyond the threshold;

(j) Load custom configuration file: specifies whether to use a user-provided file for the skeleton calibration;

- KinectDataManager: this module allows user's tracking when more than one of them are recognized by the Kinect sensor. The number of tracked users can be specified through a parameter. The module has a variable number of outputs that depends on the number of users that will be tracked simultaneously. At the beginning the outputs are not assigned to specific users; then, recognized users are sorted according to a specified criteria (e.g., label, index, distance from a given point), and each one of them is assigned to an available output. When one output is assigned to a user, the output remains reserved for that user (an ID is used to uniquely identify each user) independently from the sorting criteria. Only when the user with the given ID disappears, a new user may be assigned to the corresponding output. The assignment to an output is based on the user-specified sorting criteria, however, users already assigned to some outputs are excluded from the list of candidates. A reset command is available to remove the binding between user identifiers and output and restore the module to its initial condition. The following information is provided as output for each tracked user:

(a) Label (i.e., its unique identifier);

(b) Status with respect to the system (it can be "detected", "tracking", "calibrating", "Out of sight");

(c) 2D coordinates of the points of the skeleton (2D coordinates are normalized in the range $0.0 - 1.0$, $(0.0, 0.0)$ being the top-left corner of the image and $(1.0, 0.0)$ being the bottom-right corner;

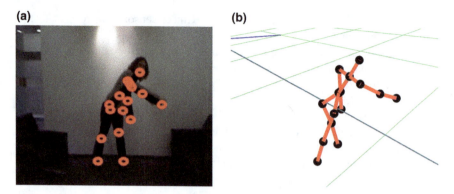

Fig. 3.2 Outputs of the tracking system. **a** 2D coordinates of the user's tracked joints drawn on live image. **b** 3D visualization of the user's tracked skeleton

(d) 3D coordinate of the points of the skeleton in normalized image coordinates or real word coordinates, according to the setting of the KinectExtractor block;

(e) Blob2D, an image containing white pixels where the user is visible in the scene, and black pixels if the corresponding pixel is not occupied by the given user.

The EyesWeb XMI platform provides a large number of modules for both 2D and 3D visualization and analysis of the captured data. The next section describes some blocks that employ data collected by the motion tracking modules to perform feature extraction and movement analysis.

3.4.2 Movement Features Extraction

Many researchers on human movement, like Wallbott & Scherer [21], Gallaher [22], deem it is important in recognizing emotions the evaluation of body motion features such as: speed, amplitude, energy and so on. Wallbott demonstrated in [23] that body activity, expansiveness and power are discriminating factors in communicating a large number of emotional states. The choreographer Rudolf Laban elaborated in his Theory of Effort [24], a model for describing expressive movement in dance.

These features address three levels of abstraction: *low, mid and high level*. The *low-level* includes features directly describing the physical characteristics of movements, such as its speed, amplitude and so on; the *mid-level* features can be described by models and algorithms based on the low-level features, for example the movement smoothness can be computed as the correlation between the movement velocity and curvature; the *high-level* features includes models that, based on a combination of low and mid-level features, describe high-level messages that can be communicated with movement, e.g., the energy flowing from the dancer's body to the audience.

In Sects. 3.4.2.1, 3.4.2.2 we define low and mid-level features that have been identified as important descriptors of Laban's high-level features described in Sect. 3.4.2.3.

3.4.2.1 Low-Level Features

As previously mentioned, Wallbott identified movement *expansiveness* as a relevant indicator for distinguishing between active and passive emotions [23]. Meijer highlighted that emotional warmth and empathy are usually expressed by open arms [25].

Wallbott also observed that the degree of movement *energy* is an important factor in discriminating emotions [23]. In his study, highest ratings for the energy characteristic corresponded to hot anger and joy while lowest values corresponded to sadness and boredom. Camurri et al. [26] showed that movement activity is a relevant feature in recognizing emotion from the full-body movement of dancers. Results showed that the energy in the anger and joy performances were significantly higher than in those expressing grief.

From the above studies we defined and implemented four low-level user's full-body movement features: the *Bounding Volume, Kinetic Energy. Bounding Ellipsoid* and *Curvature*. These features are considered a 3D extension of some previously developed 2D low-level features such as *Contraction Index* and *Motion Index* (or *Quantity of Motion*), see [27] for details.

- *Bounding Volume (BV)* - It is the normalized volume of the smallest parallelepiped enclosing the user's body. Figure 3.3 shows an example of BV computation. The BV can be considered as an approximation of the user's degree of body "openness": for example, if the user stretches her arms outside or upside the bounding volume, and so the BV Index, increases.
- *Kinetic Energy (KE)* - It is computed from the speed of user's body segments, tracked by Kinect, and their percentage mass as referred by [28]. In particular the full-body kinetic energy *KE* is equal to:

$$E_{FB} = \frac{1}{2} \sum_{i=0}^{n} m_i v_i^2 \qquad (3.1)$$

where m_i is the mass of the ith user's body segment (e.g., head, right/left shoulder, right/left elbow and so on) and v_i is the velocity of the ith segment, computed as the difference of the position of the segment at the current Kinect frame and the position at the previous frame.
- *Bounding Ellipsoid (BE)* - It is the minimum-volume ellipsoid enclosing a set of 3D points, e.g., either the points belonging to a 3D trajectory or the points associated to body parts, such as head, hands, and so on. The minimum-volume ellipsoid is computed applying Khachiyan's algorithm for rounding polytopes.

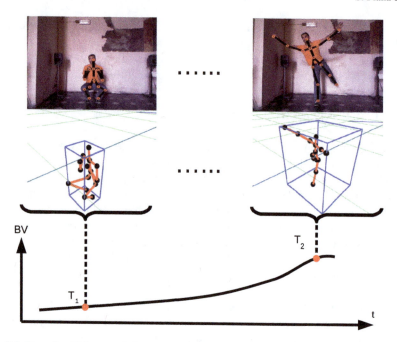

Fig. 3.3 Bounding Volume real-time computation: at time T_1 the user has a contracted posture, thus the BV value is very low; at time T_2 the user reaches an expanded posture, exhibiting a higher value for the BV

- *Curvature* (K) - It is an approximation of the curvature of a 3D trajectory: the approximation consists of computing the plane that best fits a set of 3D points within a given radius and then calculating the average distance in the points from the plane.

3.4.2.2 Mid-Level Features

- *Impulsivity Index* $(ImpI)$ - Impulsive body movements are those performed quickly, with a high energy and by suddenly moving spine/limbs in a straight direction. We adopt this definition after reviewing some literature about human movement analysis and synthesis.

  Wilson, Bobick and Cassell [29] studied *beat* gestures, those produced while accompanying speech to stress/underline the goal-conveying words during conversations, like pitch accents do for speech. Wilson and colleagues found that stroke gestures have a lower number of execution phases compared to other conversational gestures, suggesting that their execution is shorter in time.

Following the Laban theory, as described by Shapiro in [30], impulsive gestures have quick Time and free Flow, that is, they are executed quickly with energy flowing through body in a consciously uncontrolled way.

Finally, Bishko [31] defines impulsive gestures as "an accent leading to decreasing intensity".

The proposed measure for the *Impulsivity Index* mid-level feature is a combination of the two low-level features Kinetic Energy (*KE*) and Bounding Volume. *KE* is firstly used to identify the gesture duration dt: for example, using an adaptive threshold, when the *KE* becomes greater than the threshold the gesture beginning time is identified; when the *KE* goes below the threshold the ending time is identified. Then, if the *KE* is higher than a fixed energy energy threshold and the gesture length dt is lower than a fixed time threshold then Impulsivity Index is equal to the the ratio between the variation of *BV* and the gesture length dt:

let $time\_threshold = 0.45$ s;
let $energy\_threshold = 0.02$;
if $(KE \geq energy\_threshold)$ then evaluate the $GestureTimeDuration\ dt$;
if $(dt \leq time\_threshold)$ then $ImpulsivityIndex = \Delta BV/dt$;

The values of the thresholds have been evaluated through perception tests on videos portraying people who performed highly and lowly impulsive gestures, as described in [32].

• *Symmetry Index* (*SI*) - Lateral asymmetry of emotion expression has long been studied in face expressions resulting in valuable insights about a general hemisphere dominance in the control of emotional expression. An established example is the expressive advantage of the left hemiface that has been demonstrated with chimeric face stimuli, static pictures of emotional expressions with one side of the face replaced by the mirror image of the other. A study by Roether et al. [33] on human gait demonstrated pronounced lateral asymmetries also in human emotional full-body movement. Twenty-four actors (with an equal number of right and left-handed subjects) were recorded by using a motion capture system during neutral walking and emotionally expressive walking (anger, happiness, sadness). For all three emotions, the left body side moves with significantly higher amplitude and energy. Perceptual validation of the results was conducted through the creation of chimeric walkers using the joint-angle trajectories of one body half to animate completely symmetric puppets. Considering that literature pointed out the relevance of symmetry as behavioral and affective features, the symmetry of gestures and its relation with emotional expression is addressed. The *Symmetry Index SI* is measured evaluating limbs spatial symmetry with respect to the body, computing symmetry on each of the available dimensions (X, Y and Z in the case of three-dimensional data). Each partial index ($SI_{Xi}, SI_{Yi}, SI_{Zi}$) is computed from the position of the center of mass of the user and the left and right joints (e.g., hands shoulders, foots, knees) as described below:

$$SI_{Xi} = \frac{(X_B - XL_i) - (X_B - XR_i)}{XR_i - XL_i} \quad i = 0, 1, ..., n. \tag{3.2}$$

$$SI_{Yi} = \frac{(Y_B - YL_i) - (Y_B - YR_i)}{YR_i - YL_i} \quad i = 0, 1, ..., n. \tag{3.3}$$

$$SI_{Zi} = \frac{(Z_B - ZL_i) - (Z_B - ZR_i)}{ZR_i - ZL_i} \quad i = 0, 1, ..., n. \tag{3.4}$$

where X_B, Y_B and Z_B are the coordinates of the center of mass, XL_i, YL_i and ZL_i are the coordinates of a left joint (e.g., left hand, left shoulder, left foot, etc.) and XR_i, YR_i and ZR_i are the coordinates of a right joint (e.g., right hand, right shoulder, right foot, etc). The three partial symmetry indexes SI_X, SI_Y and SI_Z are then computed as follows:

$$SI_X = \frac{\sum_{i=0}^{n} SI_{Xi}}{n} \tag{3.5}$$

$$SI_Y = \frac{\sum_{i=0}^{n} SI_{Yi}}{n} \tag{3.6}$$

$$SI_Z = \frac{\sum_{i=0}^{n} SI_{Zi}}{n} \tag{3.7}$$

The three partial indexes SI_X, SI_Y and SI_Z are then combined in a normalized index that expresses the overall estimated symmetry.
- *Sphericity Index (SphI)* - Sphericity of a Bounding Ellipsoid *BE* is defined as follows:

$$\Psi = \frac{\pi^{\frac{1}{3}}(6V_p)^{\frac{2}{3}}}{A_p} \tag{3.8}$$

where V_p is the volume of the ellipsoid and A_p is the surface area of the ellipsoid.

3.4.2.3 High-Level Features

In his *Theory of Effort* [24], the choreographer Rudolf Laban points out the dynamic nature of movement and the relationship among movement, space, and time. Laban's approach is an attempt to describe, in a formalized way, the main features of human movement without focusing on a particular kind of movement or dance expression. The basic concept of Laban's theory is Effort considered as a property of movement. From an engineering point of view, it can be represented as a vector identifying the

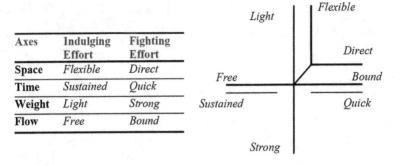

Axes	Indulging Effort	Fighting Effort
Space	*Flexible*	*Direct*
Time	*Sustained*	*Quick*
Weight	*Light*	*Strong*
Flow	*Free*	*Bound*

Fig. 3.4 The qualities of Laban's Theory of Effort. The boundaries represent opposite qualities

qualities of a movement performance. The effort vector can be regarded as having four qualities generating a four-dimensional effort space whose axes are *Space*, *Time*, *Weight*, and *Flow*. During a movement performance such an effort vector moves in the effort space. Laban investigates the possible paths followed by the vector. The expressive intentions of the movement can be associated with such paths. Each effort quality is measured on a bipolar scale, the boundaries values of which represent opposite qualities along each axis. Figure 3.4 shows the Effort's qualities and their bipolar values.

In this section, the automated extraction of high-level movement features corresponding to Laban's Effort qualities is presented. This work is part of the BeSound application developed in the framework of the EU FP7 ICT Project MIROR (Grant no. 258338, http://www.mirorproject.eu). The details of this application are out of the scope of this chapter and are described elsewhere [34].

We propose a technique, based on Support Vector Machines (SVMs), to detect 3 out of Laban's 4 Effort qualities: Time, Space and Weight.

For each quality, a set of movements were chosen following the literature and discussion with psycho-pedagogical partners of the project and with experts of Laban Movement Analysis. Then, a set of features (taken from the low and mid-level features described in Sects. 3.4.2.1, 3.4.2.2) was collected as a feature vector describing that quality.

Then, six technical recording sessions were carried out. The recordings involved six participants that were asked to mimic the selected movements. The resulting feature vectors were used to train the corresponding 3 SVMs. The output of each SVM is an integer number indicating the recognized quality and a floating-point number estimating the probability of recognition of the quality.

The RBF kernel that was used for each SVM has two parameters to be estimated: C and γ. A grid search with cross-validation was used to find the best values for C and γ: several pairs (C, γ) were tried and the one with the best cross-validation accuracy was picked. Figure 3.5 reports the best C and γ resulting from a 5-fold cross-validation. Accuracy is also shown in the fourth column of the Table.

Fig. 3.5 Values of C and γ obtaining the best accuracy for each Laban's quality

Quality	C	γ	Accuracy
Time	8.00	0.03	89.00%
Space	8.00	0.50	84.80%
Weight	128.00	0.01	99.10%

Fig. 3.6 Evaluation of the synchronization between the Kinect device and Qualisys motion capture system

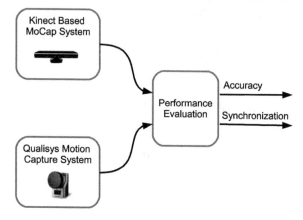

3.5 Applications

The ASC-INCLUSION project aims to create a framework, presented in Sect. 3.3, that will assist children with Autism Spectrum Conditions (ASC) and those interested in their inclusion to improve their socio-emotional communication skills. It will combine several state-of-the-art technologies in one comprehensive virtual world environment, including analysis of users' gestures, facial and vocal expressions.

The software architecture presented in Sect. 3.4 is a preliminary implementation of such technologies for detecting and analyzing nonverbal expressive body gestures relevant in the context of ASC.

A fully functional system will be achieved in the near future by performing the following macro-steps:

- firstly, algorithms will be developed for gesture segmentation, i.e., identification of significant time intervals where gesture units are performed;
- then the work will focus on the identification of the performed gesture (e.g., head shaking, greeting, ...) and on the extraction of an extended set of expressive features characterizing movement interpretation, like fluidity, repetitiveness and so on;
- automated classification of high-level expressive and emotion qualities grounded on the set of gestures and expressive features will be performed;
- finally the expressive gesture analysis modules previously implemented will be validated and adapted based on field tests with ASC children and expert observations;

Two key aspects of evaluation that are currently faced are the following: (i) the accuracy of the data tracked by the Kinect sensor, (ii) the accuracy of synchronization of the recordings in case of multimodal recordings. To address this problem, synchronized recording sessions of Kinect sensor and Qualisys motion capture system are planned. The two motion capture systems will extract data on the same set of body joints then, accuracy and synchronization will be evaluated (see Fig. 3.6). The Qualisys motion capture system is considered as a reference and both spatial and temporal accuracy of the Kinect sensor will be measured. The optical markers used by the Qualisys system will be placed on the users as close as possible to the points generated by Kinect.

Acknowledgments This research has been partially funded by the European Community Seventh Framework Programme (FP7/2007- 2013) ICT, under grant agreement No. 289021 (ASCInclusion).

References

1. O. Golan and S. Baron-Cohen, Systemizing empathy: Teaching adults with asperger syndrome or high-functioning autism to recognize complex emotions using interactive multimedia.
2. P. G. Lacava, O. Golan, S. Baron-Cohen, and B. Smith Myles, Using assistive technology to teach emotion recognition to students with asperger syndrome, *Remedial and Special Education.* **28**(3), 174–181, (May/June 2007).
3. P. G. Lacava, A. Rankin, E. Mahlios, K. Cook, and R. L. Simpson, A single case design evaluation of a software and tutor intervention addressing emotion recognition and social interaction in four boys with asd, *Autism.* **14**(3), 161–178, (2010).
4. O. Golan, E. Ashwin, Y. Granader, S. McClintock, K. Day, V. Leggett, and S. Baron-Cohen, Enhancing emotion recognition in children with autism spectrum conditions: An intervention using animated vehicles with real emotional faces, *Journal of Autism and Developmental Disorders.* **40**, 269–279, (2010). ISSN 0162–3257. URL http://dx.doi.org/10.1007/s10803-009-0862-9. 10.1007/s10803-009-0862-9.
5. S. Baron-Cohen, O. Golan, and E. Ashwin, Teaching emotion recognition to children with autism spectrum conditions, *BJEP Monograph Series II, Number 8 - Educational, Neuroscience.* **1**(1), 115–127, (2012).
6. Y. Chang, S. Chen, and J. Huang, A kinect-based system for physical rehabilitation: A pilot study for young adults with motor disabilities, *Research in developmental disabilities.* (2011).
7. Y. Chang, S. Chen, and A. Chuang, A gesture recognition system to transition autonomously through vocational tasks for individuals with cognitive impairments, *Research in developmental disabilities.* **32**(6), 2064–2068, (2011).
8. M. Raptis, D. Kirovski, and H. Hoppes. Real-time classification of dance gestures from skeleton animation. In *Proceedings of the ACM SIGGRAPH/Eurographics symposium on Computer animation* (August, 2011).
9. S. Albrektsen. *Using the Kinect Sensor for Social Robotics.* PhD thesis, Norwegian University of Science and Technology, (2011).
10. J. Leroy, N. Riche, F. Zajega, M. Mancas, J. Tilmanne, B. Gosselin, and T. Dutoit. The attentive machine: be different! In eds. A. Camurri and C. Costa, *Proceedings 4th International ICST Conference on Intelligent Technologies for Interactive Entertainment (INTETAIN 2011), LNICST 78.* Springer, Heidelberg, (2012).
11. R. Francese, I. Passero, and G. Tortora. Wiimote and kinect: gestural user interfaces add a natural third dimension to hci. In *Proceedings of the International Working Conference on Advanced Visual Interfaces*, pp. 116–123. ACM, (2012).
12. S. Cuccurullo, R. Francese, S. Murad, I. Passero, and M. Tucci. A gestural approach to presentation exploiting motion capture metaphors. In *Proceedings of the International Working*

Conference on Advanced Visual Interfaces, AVI '12, pp. 148–155, New York, NY, USA, (2012). ACM. ISBN 978-1-4503-1287-5.

13. D. Glowinski and M. Mancini. Towards real-time affect detection based on sample entropy analysis of expressive gesture. In ed. S. D. et al., *Proceedings of ACII 2011, Part I*, pp. 527–537. Springer-Verlag Berlin Heidelberg, (2011).

14. A. Camurri, G. Volpe, G. De Poli, and M. Leman, Communicating expressiveness and affect in multimodal interactive systems, *Multimedia, IEEE*. **12**(1), 43–53 (jan.-march, 2005).

15. A. Camurri, B. Mazzarino, M. Ricchetti, R. Timmers, and G. Volpe, Multimodal analysis of expressive gesture in music and dance performances, *Lecture Notes in Artificial Intelligence*. **2915**, 20–39, (2004).

16. D. Glowinski, N. Dael, A. Camurri, G. Volpe, M. Mortillaro, and K. Scherer, Toward a minimal representation of affective gestures, *Affective Computing, IEEE Transactions on*. **2**(2), 106–118 (april-june, 2011).

17. G. Varni, G. Volpe, and A. Camurri, A system for real-time multimodal analysis of nonverbal affective social interaction in user-centric media. **12**(6), 576–590, (2011).

18. D. Glowinski, M. Mancini, M. Rukavishnikova, V. Khomenko, and A. Camurri. Analysis of dominance in small music ensemble. In *Proceedings of the AFFINE satellite workshop of the ACM ICMI 2011 Conference*, Alicante, Spain, (2011).

19. A. Camurri, P. Coletta, G. Varni and S. Ghisio. Developing multimodal interactive systems with eyesweb xmi. In *Proceedings of the 2007 Conference on New Interfaces for Musical Expression (NIME07)*, pp. 302–305. ACM, (2007). URL http://doi.acm.org/10.1145/1279740.1279806.

20. Openni. URL http://www.openni.org/.

21. H. G. Wallbott and K. R. Scherer, Cues and channels in emotion recognition, *Journal of Personality and Social Psychology*. **51**(4), 690–699, (1986).

22. P. E. Gallaher, Individual differences in nonverbal behavior: Dimensions of style, *Journal of Personality and Social Psychology*. **63**(1), 133–145, (1992).

23. H. G. Wallbott, Bodily expression of emotion, *European Journal of Social Psychology*. **28**, 879–896, (1998).

24. R. Laban and F. C. Lawrence, *Effort*. (Macdonald & Evans, USA, 1947).

25. M. Meijer, The contribution of general features of body movement to the attribution of emotions, *Journal of Nonverbal Behavior*. **13**(4), 247–268, (1989).

26. A. Camurri, I. Lagerlöf, and G. Volpe, Recognizing emotion from dance movement: comparison of spectator recognition and automated techniques. **59**(1–2), 213–225, (2003).

27. A. Camurri, C. Canepa, P. Coletta, B. Mazzarino, and G. Volpe, Mappe per affetti erranti: a multimodal system for social active listening and expressive performance. (2008).

28. D. Winter, *Biomechanics and motor control of human movement*. (John Wiley & Sons, Inc., Toronto, 1990).

29. A. Wilson, A. Bobick, and J. Cassell. Recovering the temporal structure of natural gesture. In *Proc. of the Second Intern. Conf. on Automatic Face and Gesture Recognition*, (1996).

30. A. I. Shapiro. *The Movement Phrase and its clinical value in Dance/Movement Therapy*. PhD thesis, Master of Arts in Dance/Movement Therapy, MCP-Hahnemann University, (1999).

31. L. Bishko. The use of laban-based analysis for the discussion of computer animation. In *The 3rd Annual Conference of the Society for Animation Studies*, (1991).

32. B. Mazzarino and M. Mancini. The need for impulsivity & smoothness: improving hci by qualitatively measuring new high-level human motion features. In *Proceedings of the International Conference on Signal Processing and Multimedia Applications (IEEE sponsored), SIGMAP is part of ICETE -The International Joint Conference on e-Business and Telecommunications*. INSTICCPress, (2009). ISBN 978-989-674-005-4.

33. C. Roether, L. Omlor, and M. Giese, lateral asymmetry of bodily emotion expression. **18**(8), (2008).

34. G. Volpe, G. Varni, A. R. Addessi, and B. Mazzarino. Besound: embodied reflexion for music education in childhood. In *IDC*, pp. 172–175, (2012).

Chapter 4
Behaviometrics for Identifying Smart Home Residents

Aaron S. Crandall and Diane J. Cook

Smart homes and ambient intelligence show great promise in the fields of medical monitoring, energy efficiency and ubiquitous computing applications. Their ability to adapt and react to the people relying on them positions these systems to be invaluable tools for our aging populations. The most privacy protecting and easy to use smart home technologies often lack any kind of unique tracking technologies for individuals. Without a built-in mechanism to identify which resident is currently triggering events, new tools need to be developed to help determine the identity of the resident(s) in situ.

This work proposes and discusses the use of *behaviometrics* as a strategy for identifying people through behavior. By using behaviometrics-based approaches, the smart home may identify residents without requiring them to carry a tracking device, nor use privacy insensitive recording systems such as cameras and microphones. With the ability to identify the residents through behavior, the smart home may better react to the multitude of inhabitants in the space.

4.1 Introduction

"Smart homes" represent a rapidly maturing field of study as well as a looming business market. Its concepts are being applied to a wide range of medical, social and ecological issues. The vague definition of "smart home" allows for numerous implementations and variations to exist. At its core, a smart home is any living space that involves sensors, controllers and some kind of computer-driven decision

A. S. Crandall (✉) · D. J. Cook
School of Electrical Engineering and Computer Science, Washington State University,
Pullman, WA, USA
e-mail: aaron.crandall@email.wsu.edu
D. J. Cook
e-mail: djcook@email.wsu.edu

T. Bosse et al. (eds.), *Human Aspects in Ambient Intelligence*,
Atlantis Ambient and Pervasive Intelligence 8, DOI: 10.2991/978-94-6239-018-8_4,
© Atlantis Press and the authors 2013

making process. The addition of a proactive and intelligent decision maker to the aspects of home automation is what produces a smart home. With this loose definition in hand, the research, medical and business communities have been highly creative in leveraging this concept for their various needs.

The area with the greatest long-term feasibility for smart home commercialization is health care, though energy efficiency has a strong future in reducing our home's economic and ecological footprint. For the health care community, the ability to monitor older adults in their home to support "aging in place" [1, 2] is of significant interest.

Ideally, a smart home is subtle in its operation and conforms [3, 4] to the residents without detrimentally impacting their lifestyle. The system should take in information about the home environment and attempt to build models about the activities and interests of the residents. To make smart homes capable of supporting this goal, the research community has focused on building technologies for the detection of the Activities of Daily Living (ADLs) [5, 6], resident tracking [7, 8], resident identification [9], medical history building [2], social interaction [10], resident mental evaluation [11], and many others.

This work addresses methods of determining the residents' identities without a wireless tracking tag or biometric identifiers, such as facial recognition. With a single resident in the smart home this is a trivial problem, but multiple residents transform it into a serious issue. As soon as a second person (or other entity, such as a pet capable of causing sensor events) enters the smart home space, the multi-resident issue becomes critical. At this juncture, the smart home infrastructure must be designed to either function well in the face of several sources of data, or to differentiate between the sources by some means. If the system ignores the multi-resident problem, unaccounted for residents show up as noise in the data. In most cases, this noise in the data will lower the accuracy of algorithmic model building and interfere with operational quality. It will likely cause failure of high quality resident history building, preference generation, ADL detection, and many other computer generated models. Finding a means to address the multiple-resident problem remains a current and pressing issue for the smart home field.

To identify an anonymous resident using only low fidelity sensors, this research project leverages the concept of behaviometrics. Behaviometrics is the use of behavior to identify an actor among the group. These approaches hold more promise for smart home applications due to their position as ambient tools instead of obvious and intrusive ones that are common with biometrics. Examples of biometrics include facial recognition [12], body shape [13], fingerprints, and many more [14]. Conversely, behaviometrics use behaviors such as handwriting recognition [15], gait recognition [16], and computer interaction [17]. There have been few papers within the smart home field to date that use behaviometrics to identify individuals [18, 19]. New tools, when combined with the numerous data sources of a smart home system, allow the opportunity to determine a resident's identity via interaction with the smart home.

The hypothesis of this work is as follows: people have a variety of algorithmically differentiable behaviors that simple sensors can provide evidence of. The Center for Advanced Studies in Adaptive Systems (CASAS) at Washington State University (WSU) uses ubiquitous, passive and simple sensors to enroll individuals in the behaviometric system for future identification [9, 20]. Given a unique historical profile, a resident can then be re-identified in the future using behavior alone. This work introduces real world smart home testbed implementations and algorithms based on statistical models that leverage this concept of behaviometrics to accurately identify which person is generating events.

4.2 Project Research Testbed and Data Used

The data used for this project comes from a "real world" smart environment. This section describes the environment, as well as the form of the data collected and its processing for use in testing the algorithms.

4.2.1 Kyoto Research Testbed

The data gathered for this work comes from a smart home research testbed at the CASAS research facility. The *Kyoto* testbed is the primary research facility for the CASAS projects. This three bedroom apartment shown in Fig. 4.1 is part of the WSU University Housing system, and is ordinarily the home of two undergraduate students. *Kyoto* is designed to be a sensor-rich space designed for capturing as many ADLs and behaviors as possible. The left section in the image is the second story with bedrooms and the bathroom. The right side includes a living room, kitchen, and closets. The sensors are noted by rectangles and ovals, with the M### being motion detectors, L### lights, and D### doors.

Since its initial installation in 2007, this smart home testbed has undergone a series of improvements. These have primarily been software updates, but over time new sensors and interactive technologies have been deployed. These have focused on supporting the CASAS research objectives, such as early onset dementia evaluation and aging in place tools, although *Kyoto* is also used for studies regarding the associating of activities with energy consumption. This testbed has proven highly successful at gathering rich and well-documented data sets, many of which are available publicly [21].

The *Kyoto* testbed, also known as the "smart apartment" in many CASAS works, is representative of many American living spaces. Each resident has their own room with a bed, desk and closet. There is a shared bathroom, living room and kitchen. This resemblance to many typical homes makes the results from the research done here more generalizable than partial smart home implementations or work done with specialized facilities.

The sensor layout of *Kyoto* is dense, and fairly regular in design. The primary sensor type is the downward facing PIR Motion Sensor. These are installed on the

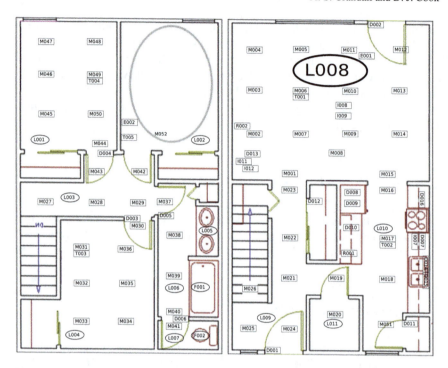

Fig. 4.1 Floorplan and sensor layout for the CASAS *Kyoto* testbed

2.4 m high ceilings with a field of view that covers roughly a 1.2 m × 1.2 m section of the floor. This sensor distribution is designed to provide enough resolution for human annotators and algorithms to localize and track the residents.

The rest of the sensors are installed on an "as needed" basis. Many of them have very specific uses to aid the artificial intelligence algorithms in their operation or to give human annotators information about the activities being performed. More detail on the *Kyoto* facility may be found in other CASAS publications [8].

4.2.2 Data Format and Annotation

The data collected from *Kyoto* was selected because it encompasses well defined times when multiple residents were occupying the space. The CASAS team did not intervene with the residents while they lived in the smart home spaces and no attempts were made to adjust their behavior over time. The residents were consulted about their behaviors to ensure an accurate final ground truth during the data annotation period.

After annotation processing, the data has five fields as shown in Table 4.1. The first four fields are generated automatically by the CASAS middleware at the time

Table 4.1 Data provided by every event, including annotation tag for person's identity

Field	Notes
Date	ISO 8601 format (yyyy-mm-dd)
Time	ISO 8601 time format (hh:mm:ss.subsec)
Serial	Unique text identifier for sensor reporting
Message	Value of sensor event
Id	Annotation tag for person causing event

Table 4.2 Example of data used for classifier training

Date	Time	Location	Message	ID
2007-12-21	16:41:41.0764	L017	ON	Res1
2007-12-21	16:44:36.8230	L017	OFF	Res1
2007-12-24	08:13:50.2819	L007	ON	Res2
2007-12-24	14:31:30.6889	L007	OFF	Res2

Table 4.3 Summary of data sets used for validation of identification algorithms

Data Set	Residents	Length	Num Events
B&B	2	5 days	20,000
TwoR	2	56 days	136,504

of the event's creation. The annotated class field is the target feature for our learning problem and contains the resident ID, to which the other fields can be mapped. An example of the data from these two data sets may be seen in Table 4.2.

The first data set, labeled *B&B*, we collected sensor data from the *Kyoto* smart apartment while two residents lived there. This data set assesses the basic ability of our algorithms to identify residents even when they occupy the space simultaneously with little training data to learn with. Both residents occupied a separate bedroom, but regularly shared the common space downstairs.

The other data set, labeled the *TwoR*, contains sensor events collected over a period of eight weeks while two residents (different than those in the *B&B* data set) lived in the *Kyoto* smart apartment. As with the *B&B* data set, this was collected to evaluate the mapping of sensor events to specific residents. However, we also used this data set to test ADL detection with other algorithms. To demonstrate the benefits of first determining the resident ID for an event on ADL detection, we performed this activity recognition first without resident identifier information and then second when the data is enhanced by adding the automatically-labeled resident identifier to each sensor event. In this manner, we determined how well residents may be recognized and the degree to which this information aids in other multi-resident tasks such as activity recognition.

4.3 Algorithms

Two algorithms were developed to test the hypothesis that behaviometrics can be used to identify individuals in a smart home space. They are based on well established machine learning algorithms and applied here to the smart home domain. Each of these tools has requirements for operation and provides unique benefits when used to identify the current residents in a smart home space. These two algorithms are:

(1) NB/ID: A naïve Bayesian-based tool
(2) HMM/ID: A Hidden Markov Model-based tool

4.3.1 Naïve Bayes: NB/ID

The first algorithm built and tested for identification was based around a Naïve Bayes classifier. In our study this tool was designated the Naïve Bayes / IDentifier (NB/ID). This classifier leverages Bayes' Rule to use the current event received to guess at the identity of the individual. Naïve Bayes classifiers have been used to good effect in other smart home contexts [22, 23]. The location, message and time features from individual events were exploited to determine the resident's identity.

A Naïve Bayes classifier uses the relative frequency of data points, their feature descriptors, and their labels to learn a mapping from a data point description to a classification label. The resident label, r, is calculated as shown in Eq. 4.1.

$$arg\ max_{r \in R}\ P(r|D) = \frac{P(D|r)P(r)}{P(D)} \quad (4.1)$$

In this calculation, D represents the feature values derived from the event to be classified. The denominator will be the same for all values of r, so we calculate only the numerator values (Table 4.3). The numerator is made of $P(r)$, which is estimated by the proportion of cases for which the resident label occurs overall and $P(D|r)$ which is calculated as the probability of the feature value combination for the particular observed resident id, or $\Pi_i\ P(d_i|r)$.

4.3.1.1 NB/ID Data Features

For a given event, the resident ID is set by the annotation process, but the feature representing that event can be derived in a variety of ways. We could attempt to use only location and message information as input to the learning problem, as shown in Table 4.4, type 1 (e.g. "Plain"), but this leaves out valuable temporal information about the resident behaviors. The remaining features, date and time, are more difficult to use. Both of these features have a very large number of possible values, so we were required to consider effective methods for abstracting date and time information.

Table 4.4 Naïve Bayes alternative time-based feature formats

Type #	Feature type	Example
1	Plain	M001#ON
2	Hour-of-Day	M001#ON#16
3	Day-of-Week	M001#ON#Friday
4	Part-of-Week	M001#ON#Weekday
5	Part-of-Day	M001#ON#Afternoon

The different feature choices that could be considered for these values, as shown in Table 4.4, divide the data in different ways and capture resident behaviors with varying degrees of fidelity.

The "Plain" feature set provides a good baseline to compare with more complex parsings. The more complex parsings, such as Part of Week (e.g. Weekday or Weekend) capture more information about the given behavior, and can furnish the classifier with more information for correct future classifications. Depending on the facets of the data set, different feature types will cause the classifier to perform better or worse.

The different feature choices available (e.g. Plain vs Hour-of-Day, etc.) divide the data up in different ways. Each method captures the behaviors or the residents with varying degrees of accuracy, depending on the feature types chosen and the behavior of the individuals in the data set.

The purely statistical nature of a Naïve Bayes classifier has the virtue of being fast for use in prediction engines, but lacks the ability to incorporate a greater context contained within the event stream that often are advantageous in discerning subtle differences in behaviors. We test the accuracy of each of these time representations when we evaluate the NB/ID algorithm.

4.3.1.2 NB/ID Summary

The statistical calculations of a Naïve Bayes classifier offer the benefit of fast learning, but lack an effective approach to reasoning about context in an event stream. In order to capture this context we also consider other approaches to learning resident IDs, as described in the next section.

4.3.2 Hidden Markov Model: HMM/ID

With this algorithm, a single model is used to encapsulate all of the residents and the sensor events they trigger. This HMM/ID tool was used to evaluate a Hidden Markov Model's ability to properly attribute events to residents.

Using the HMM, hidden nodes represent system states that are abstract and cannot be directly observed. In contrast, observable nodes represent system states that can

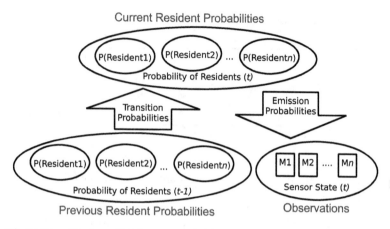

Fig. 4.2 HMM architecture of hidden states, transitions and observations

be directly observed (sensor recordings). Emission probabilities between hidden and observed nodes are learned from training data, as are transition probabilities between prior and current hidden nodes.

In our model, as shown in Fig. 4.2, each hidden node represents a single resident. The observable nodes are associated with probability distributions over feature values including the motion sensor ID and the sensor message. We can then use the Viterbi algorithm [24] to calculate the most likely sequence of hidden states that corresponds to the observed sensor sequence. This sequence of hidden states provides us with the highest-likelihood resident IDs that correspond to each sensor event in the sequence.

In the HMM/ID structure, the states Y represent the n residents from the training corpus. The start probabilities of each resident state in Y are kept in π, while the transition probabilities $a_{i,k}$ represent the likelihood of transitioning from resident Y_i to resident Y_k between events. The probability of a resident causing an event (e_t), called their emission probability, is denoted by $P(e_t|Y_i)$. If the testing corpus of sensors events is $e_0, ..., e_t$, then the state sequence $s_0, ..., s_t$ is the most likely attribution of these events to the residents represented by the states. This mapping is given by the recurrence relations in Eqs. 4.2 a–c. The result of V_t (the probabilities of all residents at event t) is the probability of the most probable series of resident attributions for the first $t-1$ events, followed by the most likely resident at time t.

$$V_0 = \forall y \in Y : P(e_0|y) \cdot \pi_y \tag{4.2a}$$

$$V_t = \forall y \in Y : P(e_t|y) \cdot \prod_{1..n}^{k} ((a_{y,Y_k}) * V_{t-1_k}) \tag{4.2b}$$

$$s_t = argmax \, V_t \tag{4.2c}$$

The events are taken one at a time without modification or manipulation, leaving the capabilities of the system entirely up to the ability of the algorithm and not choices made during pre-processing stages. The trade-off is that the tool often requires more than one event to transition between residents. It relies on some context-dependent amount of evidence for the HMM to transition from one hidden state (resident ID) to another. This sometimes leads to a delay in proper identification during operation, and is a source of error in the results. The behavior of the HMM for both "transition lag error" and "confusion error" are both discussed in Sect. 4.4.

4.3.2.1 HMM Summary

HMMs are robust in the face of noisy data and used for a number of smart home applications. The HMM/ID tool developed for classifying residents is based on a classic HMM approach and eliminates a number of shortcomings to the NB/ID tool developed earlier. This more complex algorithm reacts to the data in such a way that introduces multiple sources of error that are discussed in depth in Sect. 4.4.

4.4 Evaluation and Results

The identification algorithms introduced in Sect. 4.3 were evaluated with the data sets introduced in Sect. 4.2. The *B&B* and *TwoR* data sets are complex in nature and provide an overall evaluation of these identification tools.

Additionally, the ability for the identification results to boost ADL detection were tested with the *TwoR* data set. This test was done to demonstrate the ability for identification to provide additional features that may improve other models in the smart home context.

4.4.1 B&B Data Set Results

The *B&B* data set involves two residents simultaneously inhabiting the *Kyoto* test-bed. It is a relatively short data set of five days, but does have the benefit of being occupied nearly the full 120 h of its duration. The interleaved resident tags and the cumulative evidence for an individual's identity effecting the behavior of the NB/ID and HMM/ID models are good demonstrations of how behavior-based identification might work in a smart home context.

4.4.1.1 B&B Evaluation

The NB/ID and HMM/ID classifiers were tested using 30-fold cross validation. Each classifier was trained on 29 out of 30 groups and tested on the remaining one. The results from all 30 permutations were averaged together for an overall accuracy,

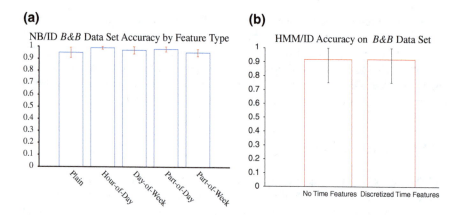

Fig. 4.3 Results for *B&B* data set. **a** NB/ID results and **b** HMM/ID results

and their variance calculated for significance values. Additional statistics showing the behavior of the classifiers and the data sets were gathered for insight into the capabilities of the tools.

The results for the tests on this data set are shown in Fig. 4.3. As can be seen, both the NB/ID and HMM/ID achieve very high classification accuracies on this two-resident, parallel-activity data. The two algorithms tested performed statistically equally on this data set. We hypothesize that having only two classes for the Naïve Bayes to choose from benefits it inordinately, at least for the behaviors exhibited by these two residents.

We found that using the Hour-of-Day gives the best results, and is a significant ($p < 0.05$) improvement over the Plain feature. Surprisingly, the inclusion of discretized time values in the HMM/ID feature vector demonstrates no benefit for the *B&B* data set. This demonstrates how both temporal and spatial information have different values for varying environments and residents. Continued efforts to discover the most valuable combination of features for identifying individuals needs to be pursued.

4.4.1.2 B&B Results Summary

The ability of our models to perform well in this unscripted, full-time, multi-resident environment is encouraging. These kinds of classifiers should be able to provide better tools for discerning an individual's activity history, even in complex multi-resident environments.

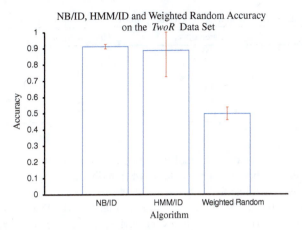

Fig. 4.4 *TwoR* data set accuracy for the NB/ID, HMM/ID and Weighted Random algorithms. The *error bars* show two standard deviations

4.4.2 TwoR Data Set Results

The *TwoR* data set provides the largest corpus of data of the three identification data sets. It has the most complex behaviors and social interactions as well. Like the *B&B* data set, the NB/ID and HMM/ID tools were evaluated for accuracy. Additionally, a more in-depth look at the behavior of the HMM/ID is discussed. Given the interleaved and social nature of the residents, the *TwoR* data exposes the various sources of error for the HMM/ID algorithm.

4.4.2.1 TwoR Evaluation

As with the evaluation of the classifiers with the *B&B* data set in Sect. 4.4.1.1, the classifiers were tested using 30-fold cross validation. Additionally, their results were compared to a Weighted Random algorithm as a base case. Each classifier was trained on 29 out of 30 groups and tested on the remaining one. The results from all 30 run permutations were averaged together for an overall accuracy, and their variance calculated for significance values. Additional statistics showing the behavior of the classifiers and the data sets were gathered for insights into the capabilities of the tools.

Both algorithms performed well on the *TwoR* and *B&B* data sets and were significantly ($p < 0.01$) better than a Weighted Random algorithm introduced as a base case for comparison. The overall accuracy of the algorithms are shown in Fig. 4.4. The HMM/ID performed slightly better than the NB/ID, though not significantly so.

Given the complexity of the data with multiple residents, and no given structure to their behavior, the highly accurate results from both algorithms attest to their robustness. Overall, the HMM/ID results are very promising. The initial hypothesis

Table 4.5 Example HMM/ID transition behavior pattern

Event number	Annotated class	Chosen class	Result
1	R1	R1	SUCCESS
2	R1	R1	SUCCESS
3	R2	R1	FAIL
4	R2	R2	SUCCESS
5	R2	R2	SUCCESS

that drawing on additional contextual information across a series of events would allow an algorithm to better differentiate between individuals seems to be supported by the overall accuracy results.

The behavior of the HMM/ID is more complex than the NB/ID when analyzing the actual pattern of classification. As the events arrive, it takes the HMM zero or more additional events to determine to whom the new events belong. For an example of this behavior, Table 4.5 shows a small snippet of events as classified by the HMM/ID. The left column is the event number, the second represents the annotated resident value for the event, the third the algorithm determined, and the final column being the success or fail results for the given event. This snippet has a transition from R1 to R2 at event #3. The HMM delays until event #4 before it has enough evidence to change states and begins attributing events correctly. This situation, where the events change from one resident to another, has been termed a resident "transition" and is an important feature of HMM/ID algorithm behavior.

By the overall accuracy metric this example has a score of 4/5, or 80 % accuracy. What is most interesting about this series is that the events arriving at the computer are initially from R1, then change to R2 at some point, but the HMM/ID algorithm takes extra events to properly transition as well. In contrast, the NB/ID algorithm takes every event in isolation, so there is no previous context to consider. With the HMM/ID algorithm, there is now a possibility of a transition window as the evidence that the new events are from a different person accumulates. The concern is that this transition window would significantly impact the effectiveness of the HMM/ID as a tool for identification.

To determine how much this transition error is effecting the HMM/ID, several statistics were gathered from the final tests. The first was the total number of occurrences in the event stream where the annotated resident value switches from one to another. This is an indication of the data complexity. If the number of transitions increases it indicates more simultaneous occupancy of the space, which can be more difficult for the HMM/ID to accurately classify.

The hypothesized inverse relationship between the rate of transitions in the data set and the final accuracy was not borne out by the results, as shown in Fig. 4.5. The transition rate line was expected to trend upward, opposite the overall accuracy across the data sets used to test the classifier. Instead it is found to trend with the accuracy, with slopes of −0.038 and −0.046 respectively. On further inspection, it is not merely the number of transitions that effects the overall accuracy, but also the location within the smart home of the residents during those transitions. If the

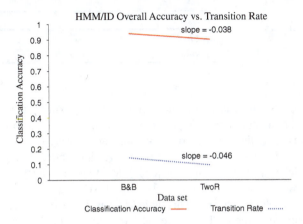

Fig. 4.5 HMM/ID's overall accuracy for each data set, with the data sets comparative transition rate. The transition rate was expected to trend opposite to the classification accuracy instead of with it

Table 4.6 HMM average transition delay length for both *B&B* and *TwoR* data sets. An average of zero would represent perfect transition accuracy

Data set	Average delay (in events)	Standard deviation (σ)
B&B	0.19	0.80
TwoR	0.38	2.17

entities' behaviors are physically close to one another, there is less evidence in the emission probabilities that the HMM should change its hidden state, and thereby transition correctly in its classifications.

If the residents are physically close together the difference in emission probabilities is lower, which causes the HMM to be less capable in detecting transitions between residents. In the *B&B* data set, the residents spent notably less time sharing communal spaces than was found in the *TwoR* data set.

As a measure of how much the delay in transition impacts the behavior of the algorithm, some additional analysis about the length of the delay was gathered. The relevant data is the average number of events after a transition before the HMM properly changes to accurately classify the resident. To find this value, the results were processed for the length of the delay in the transition on each data set.

This delay in the HMM after transitions in the data is a notable portion of the HMM's overall error. Table 4.6 shows the average length of the delay in the HMM transition for each data set. An average of zero would mean that it has no delay whatsoever on the given data set, leading to perfect classification during transitions. The lower average delay for the *B&B* data set is consistent with the overall higher accuracy as compared to the *TwoR* data set. This indicates that the HMM was able to use the evidence to accurately transition between residents based upon their behavior in the sensor space. The *TwoR* residents were notably more social than the *B&B* residents, and spent more time near one another in communal spaces during their

Table 4.7 HMM/ID
non-transition error rates

Data set	Error
B&B	3.2 %
TwoR	6.1 %

stay in the testbed. Because they spent more time in close proximity, the resolution of
the sensor network had more trouble providing evidence for the HMM to determine
who was whom during the close interactions, causing the overall accuracy to suffer.

The other sign the *TwoR* residents were more often interacting during the time of
this data gathering is the longer lengths of the HMM's transition delay. With the *B&B*
data set, there were very few instances where the HMM was not able to properly
transition within one or two events. This indicates that the residents were most often
physically separated in the testbed space. The very long delay lengths induced by
the *TwoR* were observed to be when the two residents were performing activities like
cooking or homework together. In those cases, the lack of physical separation meant
that the HMM was unable to differentiate between the residents for quite some time.

Another source of error in classification occurs when the HMM outright chooses
the incorrect class, but there was no actual transition to another resident. In this case
the algorithm is truly confused, and this error type is more akin to the type of error
in the NB/ID. The total error rate for this kind of mis-identification is summed up in
Table 4.7. The higher rate for the *TwoR* data set indicates that these two individuals
had more behavior that was similar to one another than the two people in the *B&B*
data set, which again contributes to the lower overall accuracy on the *TwoR* set.

4.4.2.2 TwoR Results Summary

Encompassing a much larger selection of behaviors over a longer time than the previous data set, the *TwoR* data set represents a valuable tool for evaluating behaviometric-
based identification algorithms. The residents are closer in behavior to one another
than those found in the *B&B* data set, which leads to more opportunities to inspect the
behavior of the algorithms themselves. These additional hurdles provide opportunity
for future identification algorithms to improve on those presented here.

4.4.3 Identification ADL Boosting

As a final demonstration of the usefulness of these identification algorithms, their
ability to aid the performance of other types of smart environment tasks needed to
be evaluated. Specifically, we apply the NB/ID classifier to the *TwoR* data set to
map sensor events to resident IDs. Given this additional identity feature, we then
use a separate Naïve Bayes classifier to identify which of 14 possible activities
the residents are individually, but concurrently performing. We evaluate the perfor-

mance of activity recognition with and without the learned resident identification to determine the extent to which the resident ID actually improves performance of our activity recognition algorithm.

The Naïve Bayes classifier initially achieved an accuracy of 80.8 % on this data set. This is a good result as compared to other published ADL detection tools, especially given the number of activities that we need to discriminate and the fact that residents are performing activities in an interwoven and parallel fashion.

To determine how activity recognition can benefit from learned resident information, we next enhance the *TwoR* data set by adding an extra field to each sensor event containing the resident ID that is automatically generated by the NB/ID classifier. We test our activity recognition algorithm again on this enhanced data set, and this time achieve an accuracy of 89.2 %. The results clearly demonstrate learned resident labels enhance the accuracy of other smart environment tasks such as activity recognition.

4.5 Conclusion

The algorithms introduced and explored in this chapter demonstrate the ability of behaviometrics to algorithmically identify smart home residents. They each leverage different aspects of the smart home data and react differently to various quantities and behaviors of residents. They are all demonstrably better than random guesses and provide additional insights into the workings of the smart home system.

The approach of using simple, passive, low resolution sensing environments with the algorithms introduced in this work generated results similar to those using other identification strategies. Controlled facial recognition approaches can see accuracies in the mid to high 1990s [25], height recognition in doorways may be 95 + % [26] and footstep and stride recognition has shown results around 87 % accurate [18]. Even RFID-based systems have some error in determining the identity of the RFID tag in real world implementations. This can lead to RFID accuracy rates of only 60–70 % [27], though repeated readings will likely overcome a single erroneous transmission. Depending upon the intended use and environment, these different approaches may have more or less utility for a given smart home installation. In the long run, some combination of available strategies will likely become the most successful behaviometric identification methods.

By applying these kinds of tools to the smart home data and generating a resident ID feature, ADL detection is boosted in complex, real world environments. Any modeling tools that improve the ability of smart homes to be functional and usable are important. Using algorithmic approaches to detect identity is a necessity for large scale deployments of smart home technologies that cannot have wireless devices affixed to every resident for identification purposes. The tools introduced and evaluated in this chapter initiate inquiry into these issues for the smart home research community.

4.5.1 Future Work

Novel approaches to behavior-based identification of actors in any system are being sought in many fields. Much of this work needs to fully define what "behavior" is, to better classify behaviometrics. For smart environments, this research should include more work on sensor selection, placement, and algorithms. Developing new tools using unsupervised learning techniques, such as Deep Belief Networks [28], will mitigate the impact of annotation requirements and lead to more deployable solutions in the future.

Acknowledgments This work was supported by the United States National Institutes of Health Grant R01EB009675 and National Science Foundation Grant CRI-0852172.

References

1. E. D. Mynatt, A.-S. Melenhorst, A. D. Fisk, and W. A. Rogers, Aware technologies for aging in place: understanding user needs and attitudes, Pervasive Computing. 3(2), 36–41 (April, 2004). doi:10.1109/MPRV.2004.1316816.
2. D. Cook, Health monitoring and assistance to support aging in place, Journal of Universal Computer Science. 12(1), 15–29, (2006). doi:10.3217/jucs-012-01-0015.
3. M. Weiser, The computer for the 21st century, Scientific American. pp. 94–104, (1991).
4. P. Rashidi and D. J. Cook, Keeping the resident in the loop: adapting the smart home to the user, IEEE Transactions on Systems, Man and Cybernetics, Part A: Systems and Humans. 39(5), 949–959 (September, 2009). doi:10.1109/TSMCA.2009.2025137.
5. V. Libal, B. Ramabhadran, N. Mana, F. Pianesi, P. Chippendale, O. Lanz, and G. Potamianos. Multimodal classification of activities of daily living inside smart homes. In eds. S. Omatu, M. Rocha, J. Bravo, F. Fernández, E. Corchado, A. Bustillo, and J. Corchado, Distributed Computing, Artificial Intelligence, Bioinformatics, Soft Computing, and Ambient Assisted Living, vol. 5518, Lecture Notes in Computer Science, pp. 687–694. Springer Berlin / Heidelberg, (2009). doi:10.1007/978-3-642-02481-8_103.
6. G. Singla, D. J. Cook, and M. Schmitter-Edgecombe, Recognizing independent and joint activities among multiple residents in smart environments, Journal of Ambient Intelligence and Humanized Computing. 1(1), 57–63, (2010). doi:10.1007/s12652-009-0007-1.
7. C. Yiu and S. Singh. Tracking people in indoor environments. In Proceedings of the International Conference on Smart Homes and Health Telematics, ICOST'07, pp. 44–53, Berlin, Heidelberg, (2007). Springer-Verlag. ISBN 978-3-540-73034-7.
8. A. S. Crandall. Behaviometrics for Multiple Residents in a Smart Environment. PhD thesis, Washington State University, (2011).
9. A. S. Crandall and D. J. Cook. Using a Hidden Markov Model for resident identification. In Proceedings of the International Conference on Intelligent Environments, IE '10, (2010).
10. D. J. Cook, A. S. Crandall, G. Singla, and B. Thomas, Detection of social interaction in smart spaces, Cybernetics and Systems: An International Journal. 41(2), 90–104, (2010). doi:10.1080/01969720903584183.
11. A. M. Seelye, M. Schmitter-Edgecombe, D. J. Cook, and A. Crandall, Smart environment prompting technologies for everyday activities in mild cognitive impairment, Journal of the International Neuropsychological Society. (2013). [To appear].
12. H. Wechsler, Reliable Face Recognition Methods: System Design, Implementation and Evaluation. International Series on Biometrics, (Springer, November 2006). ISBN 978-0-387-22372-8.

13. R. T. Collins, R. Gross, and J. Shi. Silhouette-based human identification from body shape and gait. In The Proceedings of the IEEE International Conference on Automatic Face and Gesture Recognition, pp. 366–371 (May, 2002). doi:10.1109/AFGR.2002.1004181.

14. A. K. Jain, A. Ross, and S. Prabhakar, An introduction to biometric recognition, IEEE Transactions on Circuits and Systems for Video Technology. 14(1), 4–20 (January, 2004). doi:10.1109/TCSVT.2003.818349.

15. S. N. Srihari, S.-H. Cha, H. Arora, and S. Lee. Individuality of handwriting: a validation study. In Proceedings of the International Conference on Document Analysis and Recognition, ICDAR '01, pp. 106–109, (2001). doi:10.1109/ICDAR.2001.953764.

16. C. BenAbdelkader, R. Cutler, and L. Davis. View-invariant estimation of height and stride for gait recognition. In eds. M. Tistarelli, J. Bigun, and A. Jain, Biometric Authentication, vol. 2359, Lecture Notes in Computer Science, pp. 155–167. Springer Berlin / Heidelberg, (2006). doi:10.1007/3-540-47917-1_16.

17. R. Moskovitch, C. Feher, A. Messerman, N. Kirschnick, T. Mustafic, A. Camtepe, B. Löhlein, U. Heister, S. Möller, L. Rokach, and Y. Elovici. Identity theft, computers and behavioral biometrics. In Proceedings of the IEEE International Conference on Intelligence and Security Informatics, ISI '09, pp. 155–160, Piscataway, NJ, USA (June, 2009). IEEE Press. doi:10.1109/ISI.2009.5137288.

18. R. V. Rodríguez, R. P. Lewis, J. S. D. Mason, and N. W. D. Evans, Footstep recognition for a smart home environment, International Journal of Smart Home. 2(2), 95–110 (April, 2008).

19. V. Menon, B. Jayaraman, and V. Govindaraju. Biometrics driven smart environments: Abstract framework and evaluation. In eds. F. Sandnes, Y. Zhang, C. Rong, L. Yang, and J. Ma, Ubiquitous Intelligence and Computing, vol. 5061, Lecture Notes in Computer Science, pp. 75–89. Springer Berlin / Heidelberg, (2010). doi:10.1007/978-3-540-69293-5_8.

20. A. S. Crandall and D. J. Cook. Learning activity models for multiple agents in a smart space. In eds. H. Nakashima, H. Aghajan, and J. C. Augusto, Handbook of Ambient Intelligence and Smart Environments, pp. 751–769. Springer US, (2010). doi:10.1007/978-0-387-93808-0_28.

21. W. CASAS. CASAS public smart home datasets repository. http://casas.wsu.edu/datasets.html

22. E. M. Tapia, S. S. Intille, and K. Larson. Activity recognition in the home using simple and ubiquitous sensors. In eds. A. Ferscha and F. Mattern, Pervasive Computing, vol. 3001, Lecture Notes in Computer Science, pp. 158–175, Berlin / Heidelberg, (2004). Springer-Verlag. doi:10.1007/978-3-540-24646-6_10.

23. T. van Kasteren and B. Krose. Bayesian activity recognition in residence for elders. In The IET International Conference on Intelligent Environments, IE '07, pp. 209–212 (September, 2007). ISBN 978-0-86341-853-2.

24. A. Viterbi, Error bounds for convolutional codes and an asymptotically optimum decoding algorithm, IEEE Transactions on Information Theory. 13(2), 260–269 (April, 1967). doi:10.1109/TIT.1967.1054010.

25. S. Z. Li and A. K. Jain, Eds., Handbook of Face Recognition. (Springer, March 2005), 1st edition. ISBN 978-0-38740-595-7.

26. V. Srinivasan, J. Stankovic, and K. Whitehouse. Using height sensors for biometric identification in multi-resident homes. In eds. P. Floréen, A. Krüger, and M. Spasojevic, Pervasive Computing, vol. 6030, Lecture Notes in Computer Science, pp. 337–354. Springer Berlin / Heidelberg, (2010). doi:10.1007/978-3-642-12654-3_20.

27. G. Fritz, V. Beroulle, M. Nguyen, O. Aktouf, and I. Parissis. Read-Error-Rate evaluation for RFID system on-line testing. In Proceedings of the IEEE International Mixed-Signals, Sensors and Systems Test Workshop, IMS3TW '10, pp. 1–6 (June, 2010). doi:10.1109/IMS3TW.2010.5503016.

28. G. E. Hinton. Learning multiple layers of representation. In Trends in Cognitive Sciences, vol. 11, pp. 428–434, (2007).

Chapter 5
SoundingARM Assisted Representation of a Map

Nicola Scattolin, Serena Zanolla, Antonio Rodà and Sergio Canazza

The construction of cognitive maps of spaces is fundamental for the development of orientation and mobility skills. Since the visual channel gathers most of the spatial information, people with severe visual impairments, who are partially or totally unable to see, face difficulties in: (a) moving in medium-scale spaces, where the locomotion is needed for exploration, (b) immediately recognizing the type of an indoor environment or (c) rapidly finding an object.

Assuming that the support of appropriate spatial information by means of compensatory sensorial channels may contribute to blind people's spatial performance, in this chapter we describe a non-invasive system, SoundingARM (Assisted Representation of a Map), which is able to rapidly offer an essential acoustic map of either a known and un-known indoor environment. By means of this system the user can promptly explore a room by standing at the threshold and performing a simple gesture (finger pointing). We propose the use of the Microsoft Kinect sensor to determine the user's location as well as a proprietary software that can utilize this localization data to generate vocal information about the space.

N. Scattolin (✉) · A. Rodà · S. Canazza
Department of Information Engineering, University of Padova, Padua, Italy
e-mail: nicola.scattolin@studenti.unipd.it

A.Rodà
e-mail: roda@dei.unipd.it

S. Canazza
e-mail: canazza@dei.unipd.it

S. Zanolla
Department of Mathematics and Computer Science, University of Udine, Udine, Italy

T. Bosse et al. (eds.), *Human Aspects in Ambient Intelligence*,
Atlantis Ambient and Pervasive Intelligence 8, DOI: 10.2991/978-94-6239-018-8_5,
© Atlantis Press and the authors 2013

5.1 Introduction

The ability to move autonomously in space, to recognize a place immediately, to plan a route, or to choose the shortest path is of great importance in everyday human life activities [1]. These spatial behaviors, depending on visual perception, are vital for everyone, especially for people with visual impairments who cannot—or even partially—use vision. In these cases, spatial knowledge translates into a mental representation which can normally be acquired by using supports (such as tactile maps) or constructing a cognitive map based on the direct experience of the environment [2].

The population with visual impairments can be subdivided into two groups, even though the visual impairment is a continuum that goes from severe low-vision up to no perception of light, which is to say, those with low-vision and those who are blind.

People with severe vision impairments need to use the other perceptual modalities to obtain information regarding the environment. In particular, those who are totally blind depend entirely on hearing, touch, smell in order to perceive, interact, and move about their environments [3]. The capability to independently move in space requires information-processing strategies focused, for instance, on locating objects in unfamiliar environments.

A reason to explore a room might be, for instance, to seek an object. When exploring an area, people with visual impairments usually use two specific types of independent search patterns: (a) exploration by following the perimeter which provides information on size and shape of the area and (b) exploration by means of a series of straight-line movements to and from the opposite sides of the perimeter. Once objects have been located within a space, other strategies can be adopted in order to facilitate the location of more specific objects. These strategies can be developed by walking back and forth in a straight line between two objects, or, walking back and forth between the perimeter of the area and an object. Another strategy involves using one object as a position "pin" from which straight-line paths can be made to several other objects. By means of these strategies, the user constructs a mental map, a rectangle or a braille cell, that approximates the shape of the environment and the spatial arrangement of the objects it contains [4]. Clearly all these strategies require a substantial length of time to perform locomotor exploration.

In the following paragraphs we will fully explain the SoundingARM system. In particular, in Sect. 5.2 we present the related works, whereas, in Sect. 5.3 the use of SoundingARM system, the main objectives (Sect. 5.3.1) and the requirements (Sect. 5.3.2) are introduced. Section 5.4 describes the architecture of the system in detail (the Input Components in Sect. 5.4.1, the Real-Time Processing Components in Sect. 5.4.2, the Output Components in Sect. 5.4.3, the Application in Sect. 5.4.4, and the Pure Data Patch in Sect. 5.4.5). The preliminary testing is documented in Sect. 5.5. Conclusions and future enhancements are drawn in Sect. 5.6.

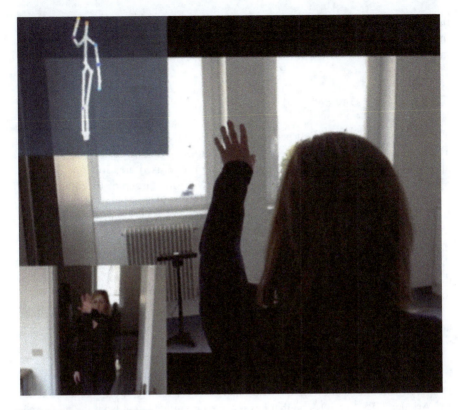

Fig. 5.1 Using soundingARM

5.2 Related Works

In the last years, the use of more and more advanced auditory display techniques has increased the possibilities to compensate the lack of vision which affects millions of blind and low-sighted people in the world. Auditory displays can aid blind people in orientation and mobility tasks.

We focus our attention on Talking Devices, from those capable of transforming texts and images into auditory information to those that allow people with visual impairments to recognize the main features of an environment.

SoundingARM (Fig. 5.1), the system presented in this chapter, can be considered a Talking Device since it aims at supplying useful spatial information by means of auditory cues (specifically, vocal information). This system, indeed, enables people with visual impairments to quickly familiarize themselves with an environment without having to perform a detailed locomotor and tactile exploration of the environment: standing at the doorway of a room and pointing in a direction with their arm, the users receive real-time text-to-speech information regarding the object placed in that direction. In this way, the user has the opportunity to build an acoustic map of the main features of the environment. This acoustic map can be used to: (a) move in space with more confidence or (b) orient oneself directly towards the object of interest.

5.2.1 Talking Devices

The aid devices for the blind people usually use speech synthesis techniques [5]. There are a lot of devices that offer information by talking to the user, first of all, the screen-reading software; the most commonly used are: Job Access With Speech (JAWS) produced by the Blind and Low Vision Group of Freedom Scientific; Window-Eyes, developed by GW Micro; VoiceOver, Apple's screen-access technology; System Access To Go (SAToGO), a free online screen-reading program for the blind and visually impaired developed by Serotek which has teamed up with the Accessibility is a Right (AIR) Foundation to offer a web-resident version of this screen reader completely free of charge; NonVisual Desktop Access (NVDA), developed by NV Access; and ZoomText, developed by Ai Squared, which allows to see and hear everything on the computer screen.

Other talking devices include reading machines, from portable to desktop solutions and computer-based to standalone solutions, which consist of a document scanner, a OCR software, and a speech synthesizer; we mention, for instance, OPENBook[1] and EYE-PAL.[2]

Recently, there are available several applications, such as Voice Brief,[3] a text-to-speech voice assistant for email and other texts for iPhone, iPod touch, and iPad and Ariadne GPS,[4] an iOs app that has received commendation from the blind and low vision community. The latter uses talking maps which allow the blind person to explore the space by moving their finger around the map. Activated VoiceOver, the app reads the street names and numbers around the user by touching them, moreover, zebra crossing are signaled by vibration. Ariadne GPS works anywhere Google Maps are available.

To extend the roundup on talking devices, we focus on "way-finding technologies" which can be subdivided into two main categories: outdoor and indoor systems. Generally, outdoor systems are based upon Global Positioning System (GPS) to locate the user: we mention, for example, the Atlas system,[5] a digital GPS-based talking map , which provides verbal information on locations, travel directions, and points of interest. Outdoor systems can rely also upon infrared communication, for instance, Talking Signs®[6] that consists of an emitter permanently installed in the environment and a hand-held receiver.

---

[1] http://www.freedomscientific.com/

[2] http://www.abisee.com/

[3] http://www.voicebriefweb.com/

[4] http://www.ariadnegps.eu/

[5] http://www.csun.edu/cod/conf/2003/proceedings/140.htm

[6] http://www.talkingsigns.com/tksinfo.shtml

The indoor systems, indeed, typically depend on infrared (IR) [6], ultrasound [7], radio frequency identifier (RFID) tags [8], or computer vision [9]. Currently, also mobile technology is delivered with applications for navigation: by combining GPS data with the data from a magnetometer, directional information can be offered to a user when the device is pointed in a specific direction [10]. In most cases the user, in order to receive spatial information, has to (a) navigate into the environment and (b) wear/hold a sensor [11].

Some way-finding systems, among those we briefly illustrated above, are very cumbersome, others foresee that the user holds pointing devices or uses a non-visual touch-screen interface; for others, the environment has to be marked with a great number of tags.

SoundingARM, unlike the systems above, does not require sensors to be worn, pointing devices to handle, or tags to mark the environment. It uses instead, standard hardware such as the Microsoft Kinect sensor and a normal Windows 7 computer; a proprietary software is used to manage the localization data in order to generate vocal information about the space. With this system, users obtain the acoustic map of the environment in a simple, fast and natural way. In the following paragraph we explain in detail how this happens.

5.3 SoundingARM (Assisted Representation of a Map)

SoundingARM, based on recognition of the user's position and movement, aims at supporting people with visual impairment in orientation and mobility tasks in known- or unknown-areas. The main aim of the SoundingARM system is to avoid, if not necessary, the locomotor/tactile exploration of an environment by giving essential spatial information: often the blind user only needs to know the environment type or whether a room contains a specific object that he/she is searching for.

Such a situation is presented to the user, for instance, when he/she enters an unknown hotel room. In this case the user immediately needs to know where the static objects are positioned in the environment (where the bed is, the bathroom, the window, etc.). The system gives an overall map of the environment that the user can then utilize to move in space with more confidence.

With SoundingARM, users need only to carry out two tasks: enter a room and, standing in the doorway, point in a direction in space with their arm (finger pointing). The system answers giving vocal information about the objects placed in that direction. These simple tasks aid blind people in developing an auditory map which can be used (1) to immediately recognize the type of environment, (2) to quickly detect a specific object, or (3) to safely move in space.

(1) Without having to wear sensors or hold pointing devices, the user, merely entering a room, receives the main information about the type of environment (kitchen, bedroom, living room); the user does not have to perform a detailed tactile activ-

ity or a locomotor exploration and does not have to learn how to manage any kind of device.

(2) If the user enters, for instance, a shop and at the entrance he/she points in a specific direction, the system provides vocal information about the type of products placed on the indicated shelves, the fixed obstacles that he/she will find on their way, and how to overcome them (in this case the user has to wear headphones).

(3) Once the information above is obtained, the user navigates with more confidence in the environment or heads straight in the right direction, saving time.

Moreover, SoundingARM allows the user to experience the environment both from an exocentric (overview, e.g. a map) and an egocentric (user-based perspective) "view" [12]. The system indeed, by using the blind user's current position data, given by the Microsoft Kinect sensor, can help them to orient themselves within the space by extracting information from the auditory map.

A demo of the SoundingARM system is available at http://youtube/VWBBihL5zbc.

5.3.1 Objectives

SoundingARM might be used with the following objectives:

- Facilitating the reintegration into private living spaces of a subject who acquired visual impairment in adolescence/adulthood.
- Encouraging the conversion of the "visual/spatial representation of space" into "an area-of-action representation of space".
- Fostering the evolution from the condition of total non-self-sufficiency through the acquisition of proficiency and safety in mobility and orientation tasks.
- Facilitating the decoding of environmental information and their organization in a spatial reference system.
- Promoting the gathering of multi-sensory information about the environment.

5.3.2 Requirements

The SoundingARM system requires:

5.3.2.1 Hardware

(1) A Microsoft Kinect sensor that detects the position of the user's arm and head thanks to a dual infrared sensor and a VGA video-camera;
(2) a PC with the following requirements:

- 15,6″, CORE I7-2670QM,

- HDD 640 GB, RAM 4 GB,
- AMD 6490M 1 GB GDDR5,
- WIN. 7 HOME. PRE. 64bit;

(3) a USB cable;
(4) two loudspeakers.

5.3.2.2 Software

(1) The Kinect for Windows software development kit (SDK) 1.0 for acquisition of Kinect data; this software allows the development of applications supporting the gesture and voice recognition;
(2) a proprietary software, developed in C++, for the management of the communication protocol with the Kinect sensor and the data relating to: (a) the user's position, (b) the measures of the room and (c) the objects;
(3) a proprietary software, developed in Pure Data, for the implementation of acoustic feedback. The basic version of SoundingARM employs a Text-to-Speech system (the speech synthesizer of Windows); the flexibility of the Pure Data platform enables us to eventually use other kinds of acoustic feedback.

5.4 The System Architecture in Detail

Figure 5.2 describes the overall system architecture of SoundingARM:

- The *Input components*: (a) a Microsoft Kinect sensor, connected by USB up to a computer with Windows 7 and (b) a configuration file, containing information about the furniture of the room; this file is loaded at the starting by the real time application.
- The *Real-time processing components*, which are: (a) the Microsoft Kinect SDK for the recognition of the skeleton, (b) the Application that analyzes the user's

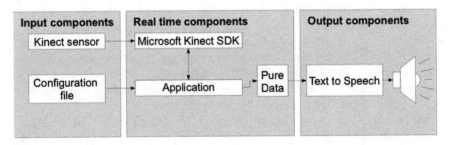

Fig. 5.2 The system architecture of soundingARM

skeleton and understands what item he/she is indicating, and (c) the Pure Data patch that works as an intermediary between the application and the text-to-speech server.

- The *Multimedia output components*: a text-to-speech server, using the Microsoft Speech API engine, gives the user a feedback of what he/she is indicating by means of stereo speakers.

5.4.1 The Input Components

The Microsoft Kinect sensor is a 3D scanner for XBOX 360. It can be also installed in a normal Windows 7 computer, thanks to the Microsoft Kinect SDK. Its drivers are developed to automatically search a human shape in an environment and calculate a fitting skeleton over the human shape. A skeleton is constituted by a collection of 3D points; every point is in relation with the joints of a person and the Kinect Sensor is at the origin of axes.

The configuration file contains information about the furniture of a room, for every object. For instance, a desk is defined as the parallelepiped that contains this object, calculating four base points, the height of the object, and the height of the object from the floor. The base points have to be taken considering the Kinect Sensor as reference system. This file contains the data of the relatively big and fixed objects of a room (for example desks, tables, wardrobe, couches) in order to give the user a spatial idea of the environment and to discern obstacles; all the moving objects (for example, chairs) are excluded and are not mapped. The application does not provide information regarding of non-static objects.

5.4.2 The Real-Time Processing Components

The Microsoft Kinect SDK contains drivers and API allowing the application to control and obtain data from the Kinect Sensor.

The kernel of the system is constituted by the Application. When it starts, it parses the configuration file initializing a data structure that represents the room furniture; after that, the configuration file is closed and the data will remain the same during all the program execution. The Application checks the presence of a human person, calculates the prospective plan of view of the room that the user should have in front of him in function of his own head position, and it checks if the user is indicating something. If the user is indicating an object, the correspondent name (in raw text format) is sent to the Pure Data patch by the Application.

The Pure Data patch has two functionalities: (a) to create a graphic user interface, in order to start and control the Application and (b) to interface the Application with the Text-to-Speech server, by using the OSC packet.

5.4.3 The Output Components

The software output component is composed by a Text-to-Speech synthesizer; it utilizes Microsoft Speech API libraries, available in Windows 7 without any installation: an English voice is installed by default; the Italian voice, necessary for the nationality of our users, is not installed. A simple way to install other voices is eSpeak, a text-to-speech application which can be used with the Microsoft Speech API.

The hardware component is constituted by two normal stereo speakers, connected to a PC via audio output jack, which reproduce the spoken version of the object textual name.

5.4.4 The Application

The Kernel is a background server Application that communicates with the Pure Data patch using the OSC packet. In loading, the Application requires a configuration file giving the room furniture data to insert into a custom read-only data structure.

After that, the Application needs for the data of the user's position to calculate his projection view. The position of the user is the position of his head joint which is available querying the Kinect drivers. When the head position is obtained, the application starts to calculate the angles that the user has to perform with his/her arms to indicate a single object. A range is obtained for every object: the minimal/maximal angle in the horizontal plane and the minimal/maximal angle in the vertical plane. The range is used to fill array cells, the indexes of the array represent the angles, whereas, the corresponding cell contains the information about the object.

In Fig. 5.3 a user is in front of a desk. He sees the desk under two range of angles, that are 75–105° and 45–70°, respectively the horizontal and the vertical

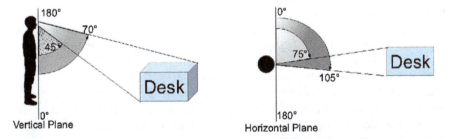

Fig. 5.3 A person is in front of a desk. On the *left* there is the representation of the user's bird's eye of the desk; on the *right* there is the representation of the user's side view. He sees this desk under an angle, whose magnitude is in function of his position in respect to desk position. This angle can be factorized in a horizontal and in a vertical component. The Vertical Plane and the Horizontal Plane are imaginary projective planes, defining the orientation of the user's view

components; in this case, the Application fills the cells in interval ([75:105], [45:70]) of the bidimensional array with the corresponding ID of the desk. The same thing is repeated for every object defined in the configuration file: the object ID is unique and consists in an increasing number, according to the position in the list of the object defined in the configuration file. The result is an integer bidimensional array of size $180 \times 180°$, that reproduces the perspective view of the room. It is updated continuously when the user moves more than 10.0 cm in every direction, that is a trade off between the accuracy of the Kinect Sensor and the recalculating costs.

The Application main aim is to understand what the user is pointing at; in order to do this it considers the hand-point and the head-point of the user. Then, it calculates the vector between the hand-point and the head-point; this vector has two angular components:

(1) the horizontal one, whose magnitude varies from the left to the right of a user with his/her view to Kinect Sensor;
(2) the vertical one, whose magnitude varies from down to up.

The horizontal and vertical angles are used as index of the bi-dimensional array, that returns the value of the object, if the user is indicating something or nothing otherwise. Supposing the user is indicating the same desk, as in the example of Fig. 5.3, the imaginary vector that joins the eyes and the left (or right) hand, must make an angle of magnitude between 75 and 105° in relation to the horizontal plane and, respectively, between 45 and 70° in relation to the vertical plane; for example, the query "array (80, 50)" will return the ID of the desk. Finally the ID is used to get the name of the selected object that is sent to the Text-to-Speech server by means of the Pure Data patch.

5.4.5 The Pure Data Patch

The Application, using OSC packet standard, transmits all the useful data to a Pure Data patch that allows the development of several types of future tools; Pure Data has been chosen for its versatility and its modularity; furthermore, it is more simple than native C++ by which the Application was written. The OSC standard does not preclude the use of other applications, similar or different to Pure Data.

Currently, the patch transmits the name of the selected object to the text-to-speech synthesizer. However, in the future, a system for rendering a 3D space using audio signals will be added; in order to do this, the patch and the Application have been already adapted: the Application is able to send to the Pure Data patch all the information about the selected object (its position and dimensions) and the position of the user. All these data are necessary to have a feedback for rendering 3D audio effects.

In addition, the Pure Data patch provides a control interface to manage the server applications; in detail, it authorizes (a) the starting of the Application and the text-to-speech synthesizer, (b) the start/stop of skeleton recognition, and eventually (c) the programs killing. In order to start executable files, the patch uses

Createprocess, a specific external function that permits the background execution of a Windows 7 application by simulating a double click in an execution file without preemption and the opening of unsightly terminal windows.

5.5 Preliminary Testing

The SoundingARM system, on March 6, 2012, was tested with ten adults with different degrees of visual disability. Some of them had also motor/cognitive impairments associated. The preliminary usability test was informal/qualitative and carried out in a kitchen of the Regional Institute "Rittmeyer" for the Blind (in Trieste, Italy). This environment was unknown to the majority of them. The overall purpose of the preliminary testing was to verify if the SoundingARM system performs at an acceptable level for these representative users. It is necessary, indeed, that the system firstly be tested by the users in order to ensure that they have a positive and efficient experience in using it.

Identified testing participants received instructions prior to the beginning of preliminary testing in order to have them familiarize with the tasks. One by one, the users were asked to: enter the room and, standing in the doorway, point the arm in several directions in order to identify the static objects. They had to identify twelve static objects; a table, a fridge, a wall cupboard, a dish-rack, an extractor fan, a cooker, a sink, a switch, two radiators, and two windows. Test-takers did not know how many objects they had to localize.

The following remarks were collected by means of the test-takers' direct observation in order to obtain information about (a) their approach to the system (their actions, potential difficulties, comments) and (b) the system performance. Even if all the test-takers identified many objects of the kitchen and enjoyed the experience, we observed that:

(1) In the first approach with the system, blind users with associated severe cognitive impairments have requested: (a) further verbal explanations compared to those scheduled, (b) a "physical guide", given that the pointing gesture has to be as precise as possible, and (c) a tactile signal on the floor in order to maintain the position on the doorway (they tend to enter the room as they do usually). Given the short duration of the initial familiarization with the system, these users were allowed to ask for help in order to perform the proper movement; in fact, they were guided by an external operator whose body however interfered with the user's skeleton recognition, leading SoundingARM to make errors.

(2) Blind test-takers, using the wheelchair, did not localize all the static objects; in these cases the system had difficulties in providing the user with all the acoustic feedback; this probably occurred because wheelchairs constituted an obstacle for the recognition of the skeleton and the head reference point was almost on the same level of the Microsoft Kinect sensor.

(3) Blind test-takers with no other associated impairment have easily identified all
     the objects of the room.

Generally, early blinds never localize any target (acoustic or not) by pointing to it,
an action related more to vision than to hearing/touch [13]. The lack of early visual
experience disturbs allocentric pointing in early congenitally blind; nevertheless,
in adulthood they fulfill pointing tasks appropriately, since over time they acquire
long-term experience without vision (e.g. to avoid static and dynamic objects in
locomotor space) [14].

   Moreover, for blind persons finger pointing is an important communication task in
interpersonal communication, in fact, it is taught in orientation and mobility courses.
The SoundingARM system, in this case, can represent a useful tool to improve this
ability. Therefore, blind persons, especially those who have cognitive impairments
associated, need for a longer period of training in order to become more accurate at
pointing[15].

   Moreover, when trying to reach a sonorous object, a blind person usually gropes
for it rather than reaching for it directly [13]. In fact, the ability to reach a specific point
directly is very difficult to acquire without visual reference points. The development
of this important ability is obtained by means of the construction of a cognitive map,
a spatial mental model [3] which, in this context, is fostered by the acoustic feedback
given by the SoundingARM system.

   Overall feedback regarding SoundingARM was positive (informal interview).
All participants indicated that they would enjoy using the system and that their
performance would improve with more time to practice using it.

5.6 Conclusions and Future Enhancements

SoundingARM is a pointing-based system which aims at allowing users with severe
visual impairments to build a spatial mental map of an unknown indoor environment.
The subject has the possibility of constructing a cognitive map of the environment
by means of the acoustic feedback provided by the system. This spatial map may be
used (a) to immediately recognize the type of indoor environment, (b) to confidently
move in space, or (c) to quickly detect a specific object.

   With SoundingARM, blind users, entering an unknown room, need not immediately perform the locomotor exploration or tactile activity since the system provides
vocal information which allows them to "acoustically discover" the main features of
the environment and the objects in it. The users, by performing a simple and bounded
gesture (finger pointing), receive from the system several spatial affordances (household sounds).

   The spatial orientation and mobility tasks can be facilitated by the speech information on the placement of static objects, given by the system. At the same time,
the user employs the motor information deriving from the arm position to obtain the
spatial data necessary for the objects localization.

Some software improvements have to be implemented to make the application more stable in particular for users in wheelchair and for multi-user contexts. The problem of the interference on the part of an external operator (during the training path) can be solved adding a multi-user management to the system. In the future it might also be possible to enhance the system by adding the spatialization of sound events in order to offer the user a complete spatial information about the location of the objects.

Improvements of the system, in order to enable the recognition (e.g. by means of video-signal processing techniques) of semi-static objects or other things that can easily be moved but normally remain in the same room, are possible but not part of our short-term objectives. Our main interest, in fact, is to investigate if and to which extent the gestural interaction, on which SoundingARM is based, is effective in fostering the construction of a spatial map of unknown indoor environments. With this aim we will conduct an experimentation with which we intend to assess: (a) if the representation is actually established and the space is well understood by means of fixed stimuli and without interaction and (b) how the interaction improves the acquisition of the spatial representation.

However, the main function of SoundingARM—the recognition of the pointing gesture—is fully satisfactory and the results obtained are encouraging.

Acknowledgments This work has been partially supported by the Regional Institute "Rittmeyer" for the Blind of Trieste (Italy) through the project "*Evoluzione dei sistemi di feedback acustico per la prima domiciliazione dei soggetti con inabilità visiva acquisita*" (Evolution of acoustic feedback systems for the homecoming of subjects with acquired vision impairment) funded by Friuli Venezia Giulia Region (Italy), Decree n. 1265/AREF dd. November 25th, 2010.

References

1. S. Zanolla, F. Romano, F. Scattolin, A. Rodà, S. Canazza, and G. L. Foresti. When sound teaches. In eds. S. Zanolla, F. Avanzini, S. Canazza, and A. de Götzen, *Proceedings of the SMC 2011–8th Sound and Music Computing Conference*, pp. 64–69, (2011).
2. C. Thinus-Blanc and F. Gaunet, Representation of space in blind persons: Vision as a spatial sense?, *Psychological Bulletin*. **121**(1), 20–42, (1997).
3. Y. Hatwell, *Psicologia cognitiva della cecità precoce*. (Biblioteca Italiana per i Ciechi "Regina Margherita"- ONLUS, 2010).
4. E. W. Hill and J. J. Rieser, How persons with visual impairments explore novel spaces: strategies of good and poor performers., *Journal of Visual Impairment and Blindness*. **87**(8), 295 (October, 1993).
5. R. W. Massof. Auditory assistive devices for the blind. In *Proceedings of the International Conference on Auditory Display*, pp. 271–275, Boston, MA, USA (July, 2003).
6. Y. Sonnenblick. An indoor navigation system for blind individuals. In *Proceedings of the 13th annual Conference on Technology and Persons with Disabilities*, (1998).
7. L. Ran, S. Helal, S. Moore. Drishti: An integrated indoor/outdoor blind navigation system and service. In *IEEE International Conference on Pervasive Computing and, Communications*, (2004).
8. S. Mau, N. A. Melchior, M. Makatchev, and A. Steinfeld, *BlindAid: An Electronic Travel Aid for the Blind*. 2008.

9. A. Hub, J. Diepstraten, and T. Ertl, Design and development of an indoor navigation and object identification system for the blind, *SIGACCESS Access. Comput.* (77–78), 147–152, (2004).
10. C. Magnusson, M. Molina, K. Rassmus-Gröhn, and D. Szymczak. Pointing for non-visual orientation and navigation. In *Proceeding of NordiCHI, Reykjavik, Iceland* (October, 2010).
11. A. Fusiello, A. Panuccio, V. Murino, F. Fontana, and D. Rocchesso. A multimodal electronic travel aid device. In *Proceedings of ICMI*, pp. 39–46, (2002).
12. R. Ramanathan, Combining egocentric and exocentric views: enhancing the virtual worlds, interface. 1999.
13. M. C. Wanet and C. Veraart, Processing of auditory information by the blind in spatial localization tasks, *Perception and Psychophysics*. (38), 91–96, (1985).
14. M. Ittyerah, F. Gaunet, and Y. Rossetti, Pointing with the left and right hands in congenitally blind children, *Brain and Cognition*. **64**, 170–183 (April, 2007).
15. S. Zanolla, A. Rodà, F. Romano, F. Scattolin, G. L. Foresti, S. Canazza, C. Canepa, P. Coletta, and G. Volpe. Teaching by means of a technologically augmented environment: the Stanza Logo-Motoria. In *Proceedings of INTETAIN 2011 Conference*, (2011).

Part III
Lifestyle Support

Chapter 6
Ambient Support by a Personal Coach for Exercising and Rehabilitation

Maarten F. Bobbert, Mark Hoogendoorn, Arthur J. van Soest, Vera Stebletsova and Jan Treur

In this chapter an agent-based ambient system is presented to support persons in learning specific movement patterns. The ambient system serves as a personal coach that observes a person's movement pattern, and analyses this based on comparison with an ideal pattern generated by optimisation using a computational musculoskeletal model for this type of pattern minimizing knee joint loading. Based on this analysis the Personal Coach generates advice to adapt the person's pattern in order to better approximate the ideal pattern. The Personal Coach has been designed using the agent design method DESIRE, thereby reusing an available generic agent model. The system was evaluated (a proof of principle) by setting up an environment in which sensoring of body part positions was incorporated. In evaluations with a few subjects substantial improvement of the movement pattern compared to the ideal movement pattern was achieved.

M. F. Bobbbert · A. J. van Soest
Faculty of Human Movement Sciences, VU University, Amsterdam, The Netherlands
e-mail: m.f.bobbert@vu.nl

A. J. van Soest
e-mail: a.j.van.soest@vu.nl

M. Hoogendoorn · V. Stebletsova · J. Treur (✉)
Faculty of Exact Sciences, Agent Systems Research Group, VU University, Amsterdam,
The Netherlands
e-mail: j.treur@vu.nl

M. Hoogendoorn
e-mail: m.hoogendoorn@vu.nl

V. Stebletsova
e-mail: v.n.stebletsova@vu.nl

T. Bosse et al. (eds.), *Human Aspects in Ambient Intelligence*,
Atlantis Ambient and Pervasive Intelligence 8, DOI: 10.2991/978-94-6239-018-8_6,
© Atlantis Press and the authors 2013

6.1 Introduction

Within the area of exercising and rehabilitation, personal coaching can be a crucial factor for success. This holds in particular when patterns of movements have to be learned which are quite complex, or which are hard to perform due to limitations of the person, as in rehabilitation. Only trying the same type of movement pattern over and over again, thereby hoping to learn from experience, may be a very long way to a desired situation or may not even lead to a desired situation at all. Personal feedback from a coach may be essential to make substantial progress. However, giving such feedback is far from trivial, as it has to be well-informed. In the first place a coach has to monitor very well the exact movements over time from the person, where very small differences in timing may already be crucial. In the second place a coach needs knowledge about how the movement pattern can be optimal. Finally, a coach has to be able to point out how the monitored pattern can be changed towards an optimal pattern, by giving important suggestions without overloading the person.

As pointed out above a coach needs to fulfil rather demanding requirements: in observation capabilities, in having knowledge about movement patterns, and in the interaction with the person. Ambient Intelligence is an area in which such types of capabilities needed for personal support are incorporated in the environment in an automated manner; see, e.g., Aarts, Harwig, and Schuurmans [2], Aarts and Grotenhuis [1]; Riva, Vatalaro, Davide, and Alcañiz [18], Sadri [19]. For example, observation capabilities can be realised using sensor systems, and domain knowledge may be made available in the form of computational models of the human processes considered; e.g., Treur [20], Bosse, Both, Gerritsen, Hoogendoorn, Treur [5].

This chapter presents an architecture of a personal coach for exercising and rehabilitation and its application to teaching persons a specific target movement pattern to stand up from a chair (henceforth referred to as sit-to-stand, STS, movement; e.g., Doorenbosch, Harlaar, Roebroeck, Lankhorst [11], Janssen, Bussmann, Stam [15], Yoshioka, Nagano, Himeno and Fukashiro [25], De Morree [10], Winter [24]. The architecture has been designed as a specialisation of the personal assistant agent model described by Bosse, Hoogendoorn, Klein, and Treur [6], using the agent design method DESIRE; cf. Brazier, Jonker, and Treur [8]. The specific target STS movement was obtained using movement simulation (Casius, Bobbert, Soest [9]): the motion of a musculoskeletal model was optimized to minimize the peak knee joint moment reached during the movement. Finally, persons were coached to approximate this optimal STS movement using monitored kinematics and ground reaction forces. In the end it was checked whether the peak knee joint moment of the persons had indeed become smaller after coaching).

6.2 Overview of the Overall Method Used

The method used involves observing a movement pattern by observation and comparing that with an ideal pattern. The movement pattern is described by values for a number of relevant variables considered over the time period of the exercise. Examples of variables are the positions of hip, knee, ankle, toe that can be observed, forces that are exerted, and information that can be derived from this such as angles between different parts of the body, and movement speeds. Let the vectors $\underline{op}(t)$ and $\underline{ip}(t)$ for each time point t within the exercise be defined by

$\underline{op}(t)$ the person's observed movement pattern
$\underline{ip}(t)$ the ideal movement pattern

The components of these vectors are the values at t of the relevant variables considered. The values of these vectors are determined as follows. For $\underline{op}(t)$ at a number of points on the body LED markers are attached (e.g., on knee, ankle, hip, toe) that can easily be tracked over time by sensors. Moreover, sensors are used to measure forces exerted on the ground. This sensor information is acquired by the ambient system and stored. The values of the ideal movement pattern are determined by optimising the pattern based on a computational musculoskeletal model. The *deviation pattern* $\underline{d}(t)$ is the difference vector

$$\underline{d}(t) = \underline{op}(t) - \underline{ip}(t)$$

This indicates the deviation of the observed pattern from the ideal pattern. For each time point t within the exercise period in principle a possible advice is to make the difference between observed and ideal pattern at that time point t smaller by $\underline{d}(t)$, i.e., by making the new movement pattern $\underline{op}'(t)$ as follows:

$$\underline{op}'(t) = \underline{op}(t) - \underline{d}(t) = \underline{op}(t) - (\underline{op}(t) - \underline{ip}(t)) = \underline{ip}(t)$$

Such an advice could be formulated as: at t change all the positions by $\underline{d}(t)$. However, giving all this advice for all time points t and for all components of the vector would not be realistic. It simply would be too much for the person to follow all this advice. Therefore an important capability of a personal coach is to determine in an intelligent manner a *focus advice set*, which is a limited subset of the set of all possible advice options. The idea is that such a focus advice set can be determined based on one or a number of criteria values $c_i(t)$ for the possible advice options. Examples of such criteria are listed below. Note that these are high-level specifications to get an intuition for such criteria. Here the considered time interval is the execution of the exercise (sit-to-stand):

- *single versus multiple correction*

  - indicated by a number between 0 (single) and 1 (all)
  - 'single' means per time point only one position (e.g., knee position) is corrected
  - 'multiple' means per time point more positions (e.g., knee, ankle and toe position) are corrected

- *wide versus narrow*

  - indicated by a number between 0 (narrow) and 1 (wide)

- 'narrow' concentrates on the points in time with highest deviations
- 'wide' addresses all deviations

- *early versus late*

  - indicated by a number between 0 (early) and 1 (late)
  - 'early'concentrates on the early part of the time axis
  - 'late' concentrates on the later part of the time axis
  - for example, 0.5 concentrates on the middle area

- *causes versus consequences*

  - if a deviation is noticed, this may be the consequence of some cause earlier in time; it may be preferable to take such a cause as point of correction, and not the consequence and assign a number accordingly.

- *threshold*

  - indicated by a number between 0 (low threshold) and 1 (high threshold)
  - only the possible advice options are chosen for which the deviation divided by the maximal deviation is above the threshold.

To define the focus advice set, one of these criteria $c_i(t)$ can be chosen, or a subset of them. In the latter case it can be useful to use weight factors and determine an aggregated criterion value by a weighted average $aggc(t) = \Sigma w_i c_i(t)$, and only choosing the possible advice options with this value above a certain threshold τ: aggc(t) $>\tau$. Such weight factors can be chosen equal by default, or, for example, based on expert knowledge from experienced therapists, differences can be made.

6.3 Finding the Ideal Movement Pattern for the STS Task

In this section it is briefly described how the ideal movement pattern $ip(t)$ was determined for the STS task by using a numerical musculoskeletal model and optimisation techniques.

Musculoskeletal model

For simulation of the STS task a two-dimensional forward dynamic model of the human musculoskeletal system was used; cf. van Soest, Schwab, Bobbert, van Ingen Schenau [23]. The model (see Fig. 6.1), which had the time-dependent muscle stimulation *STIM* as its only independent input, consisted of four rigid segments representing feet, shanks, thighs and HAT (head, arms and trunk). These segments were interconnected by hinges representing hip, knee, and ankle joints, and the distal part of the foot was connected to the ground by a hinge joint. Nine major muscle-tendon complexes (MTC) of the lower extremity were embedded in the skeletal model: m. gluteus maximus, biarticular heads of the hamstrings, short head of m. biceps femoris, m. iliopsoas, m. rectus femoris, mm. vasti, m. gastrocnemius, m.

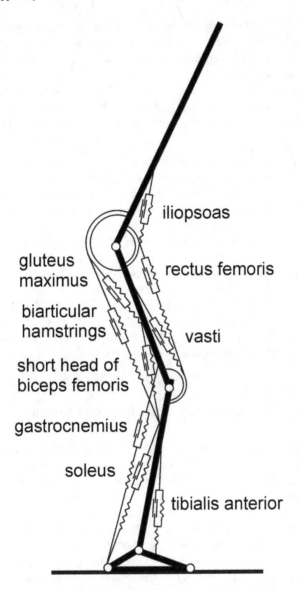

Fig. 6.1 Model of the musculoskeletal system used for forward dynamic simulations. The model consisted of four interconnected rigid segments and nine muscle–tendon complexes of the lower extremity, all represented by Hill type muscle models. The only input of the model was muscle stimulation as a function of time

soleus and m. tibialis anterior; cf. Bobbert and Casius [4]. Each MTC was represented using a Hill-type unit. The MTC model, which has also been described in full detail elsewhere (van Soest and Bobbert [21]) consisted of a contractile element (CE), a series elastic element (SEE) and a parallel elastic element (PEE). Briefly, behaviour of SEE and PEE was determined by a simple quadratic force-length relationship, while behavior of CE was complex: CE velocity depended on CE length, force and active state, with the latter being defined as the relative amount of calcium bound to troponin (Ebashi and Endo [12]).

Following Hatze [14] the relationship between active state and *STIM* was modelled as a first order process. *STIM*, ranging between 0 and 1, was a one-dimensional representation of the effects of recruitment and firing frequency of α-motoneurons.

Optimisation

The model was put in a standard static initial posture to stand up from a chair, and had to achieve a postureclose to a fully extended standing position, while joint angular velocities were close to zero. For the application in this chapter, the ideal motion was defined as the motion for which the peak knee extension moment was minimal while satisfying the constraints mentioned above.

To achieve this, an objective function as described elsewhere was defined (Bobbert and Casius [4]), incorporating penalties on deviations from the desired final configuration, and the peak knee extension moment. Then the objective function was minimized by optimizing for each of the muscles four instants at which *STIM* changed and for each of these the piecewise constant *STIM*-level to which the change occurred. For the optimization, a parallel genetic algorithm was used (van Soest and Casius [22]). The motion pattern corresponding to the optimal $STIM(t)$ solutions was used as the ideal motion pattern $\underline{ip}(t)$.

6.4 The Agent Architecture for the Personal Coach

In this section an overview is given of a dedicated generic agent model that can be used as a Personal Coach for performing and training for physical exercising and rehabilitation. It will be illustrated for the process of standing up from a chair as part of a rehabilitation process. The agent uses a computational model of the supported physical process to obtain an ideal way of performing the exercise, as described in Sect. 6.2. Moreover, it uses information of the human actually performing the exercise obtained by monitoring (for more details, see Sect. 6.6), in order to analyse what still has to be improved, and to determine which aspect is brought under the attention of the human as an intervention. The model was specified using the component-based agent system design method DESIRE (DEsign and Specification of Interacting REasoning components; cf. Brazier, Jonker and Treur [8]) and automatically implemented using the DESIRE software environment, and in a dedicated Matlab version. Below the design of the model is described by the interacting components at different levels of process abstraction. Moreover, for each of the components the generic information types are described that define their input and output.

The process of standing up from a chair, used as an illustration, is monitored by the locations over time of different points of the body, and by forces exerted on the ground. Learning to stand up in the right way can be an important aspect in

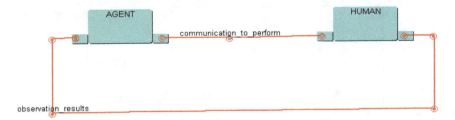

Fig. 6.2 The agent system: interaction between personal coach agent and human

rehabilitation, for example, to avoid pain and prevent old injuries from coming back. At the top level the agent system consists of two interacting agents: the human, and the Personal Coach, also called agent; see Fig. 6.2. Here, the big boxes represent components of the system whereas the small boxes and the left and right hand side represent the component input and output respectively. Note that this picture was generated by the DESIRE software environment; the same holds for Figs. 6.3, 6.4, 6.5, 6.6. The interaction between the two is modelled by means of (1) communication taking place from Personal Coach to human, but not in the opposite direction, and (2) the agent observing the human (but not the other way around). Extensions of the model could be made involving also communication from human to agent and observation of the agent by the human.

However, the model is kept simple for the purpose at hand. The following describes the generic input and output information types for both components, by showing the generic template for basic statements (atoms) that are used. Examples of instances

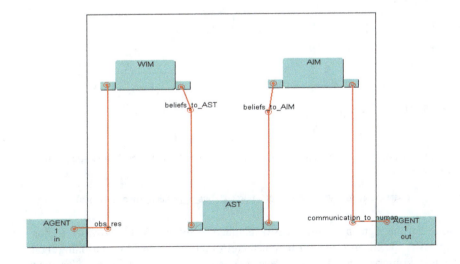

Fig. 6.3 The internal agent model used for the personal coach agent

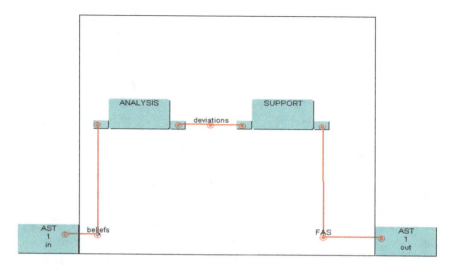

Fig. 6.4 The agent specific task as composed of an analysis and support component

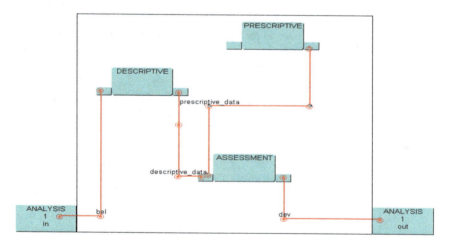

Fig. 6.5 Analysis component

for the case addressed are the following. It is observed that at time 1 the knee position of person1 is 0:

observation_result(personal_info(1, person1, has_x_position, knee, 0.0), pos)

Note that the sign (*pos* in this case) included in the predicates provides a more expressive specification of information, thereby for instance enabling reasoning about unknown observations, this is however beyond the scope of this paper. The focus

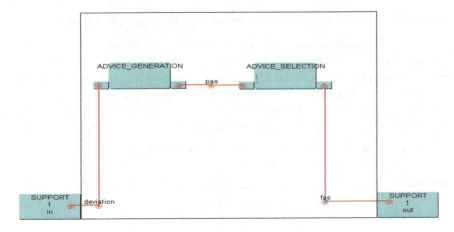

Fig. 6.6 Support component

advice for person1 to change at time 1 the knee x-position by 1 is communicated by the Personal Coach agent (note that the predicate fa stands for focus advice):

communicated_by(fa(personal_info(1, person1, has_x_position, knee, 1.0), pos, agent)

When looking inside the agent (the box at the left hand side in Fig. 6.2), a further structure is found as shown in Fig. 6.3.

For the internal design of the Personal Assistant the Generic Agent Model GAM is reused (Brazier, Jonker, and Treur [7]), from which for the moment the following three components are adopted (see Fig. 6.3):

- *World Interaction Management (WIM)*

  – handling incoming observation information (about the human performance).

- *Agent Interaction Management (AIM)*

  – handling outgoing communication (advice).

- *Agent Specific Task (AST)*

  – to determine the advice to be given.

Observations and communications as transferred internally are represented as shown above. Beliefs are transferred from World Interaction Management to AST and from AST to Agent Interaction Management. They are represented as follows. It is (positively) believed that at time 1 (within the exercise period) person1 has the knee at x-position 0:

belief(personal_info(1, person1, x-position, knee, 0), pos)

It is believed that a focus advice is to change person1's knee x-position by 1:

belief(fa(personal_info(1, person1, x-position, knee, 1)), pos)

The components Agent Interaction Management and World Interaction Management can be kept simple. Within World Interaction Management information is extracted from incoming observation results, and incorporated in beliefs. To achieve this in a general manner the following generic knowledge base element can be used, where T:TIME indicates the point of time within the exercise:

if   observation_result(personal_info(T:TIME, A:AGENT, A2:ATTRIBUTE,
        B:BODY_PART, V:VALUE), S:SIGN)

then belief(personal_info(T:TIME, A:AGENT, A2:ATTRIBUTE, B:BODY_PART, V:VALUE), S:SIGN)

Within Agent Interaction Management communications are generated based on beliefs, using the following generic knowledge base element:

if   belief(fa(personal_info(T:TIME, A:AGENT, A2:ATTRIBUTE, B:BODY_PART, V:VALUE)), pos)

then to_be_communicated_to(fa(personal_info(T:TIME, A:AGENT, A2:ATTRIBUTE,
        B:BODY_PART, V:VALUE), pos, human)

6.5 Analysis and Support Within the Agent Specific Task

Adopting elements of the reusable model presented by Bosse, Hoogendoorn, Klein, and Treur [6], within the Agent Specific Task two subtasks were modelled (see Fig. 6.4):

- *Analysis*

  – To analyse a performance by the human

- *Support*

  – To determine the support to be provided

The information transferred as output from Analysis to input for Support is of the following form.

belief(deviation(T:TIME, A:AGENT, A:ATTRIBUTE, B:BODY_PART, V:VALUE),pos)

An example instance is

belief(deviation(0, human, has_x_position, toe, 1.0), pos)

The analysis component is composed of three components:

- *Descriptive Information Maintenance*

  – Here beliefs on the human's observed current performance are determined (the vector representing the observed movement pattern $op(t)$).

- *Prescriptive Information Determination*

- Here beliefs on the ideal performance are determined (the vector representing the ideal movement pattern $\underline{ip}(t)$).

• *Assessment*

- Here assessments are done by comparing input from the two other components (determining the deviation vector $\underline{d}(t)$).

The latter component makes assessments of the performance of the human by comparing input from two other components providing, respectively *descriptive* information (beliefs on the observed current performance) and *prescriptive* information (beliefs on the performance considered as ideal); see Fig. 6.5.

An example instance of output of Assessment is

belief(deviation(0, person1, has_x_position, toe, *1.0*),pos);

which describes that at time 0 the toe is deviating from the ideal horizontal position by 1.0. Such output can be generated in Assessment by using the following simple generic knowledge base element:

if   belief(personal_info(T:TIME,idealperson,A:ATTRIBUTE,B:BODYPART,V1:reals),pos)

and belief(personal_info(T:TIME,person1,A:ATTRIBUTE,B:BODYPART,V2:reals),pos)

and V3:reals = V1:reals - V2:reals

then belief(deviation(T:TIME,person1,A:ATTRIBUTE,B:BODYPART,V3:reals),pos)

The component Support receives information about deviations for different body parts at different time points, and determines what advice should be given. Here some strategic choices have to be made, as it will not be very helpful to provide the human with an overwhelming amount of information. The process to determine the advice is composed of two subcomponents (see Fig. 6.6):

• *Advice Generation*

- providing possible advice options based on deviation information.

• *Advice Selection*

- Providing focus advice options as a limited subset of the set of possible advice options.

For the moment the choice has been made to keep the component Advice Generation simple: for every deviation identified a possible advice (to compensate the deviation) is generated. This was specified by the following generic knowledge base element in Advice Generation:

if   belief(deviation(T:TIME,person1,A:ATTRIBUTE,B:BODYPART,V1:reals),pos)

then belief(pa(T:TIME,person1,A:ATTRIBUTE,B:BODYPART,V1:reals),pos);

The component Advice Selection models a more complex process. Within Advice Selection a form of filtering of the many possible advice options is performed. To this end it is composed of two components (see Fig. 6.7):

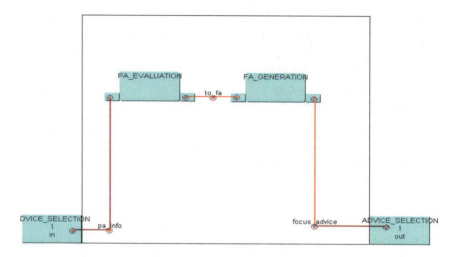

Fig. 6.7 Advice selection component

- *Possible Advice Evaluation*
    - where each possible advice is valuated (rated between 0 and 1) for a number of criteria.
- *Focus Advice Generation*
    - where based on the rates of the possible advice options a selection of advice options is made (represented by the link fas).

Examples of criteria for which ratings can be determined within Possible Advice Evaluation are:

- *early or late time points of the advice*
    - Early provides high ratings for possible advice options for the early part of the time axis (which represents time of the movements), late concentrates on the later part of the time axis.
- *higher deviations*
    - Provides high ratings for possible advice options with highest deviations, and low ratings for those with low deviations.
- *longer times of deviations*
    - Provides higher ratings for possible advice options with deviations above a certain value that last long.

Rating for such criteria can be specified as part of the knowledge base of Possible Advice Evaluation, for example, as follows (here c0 is the first example criterion indicated above, and c1 the second); note that T:TIME represents the time point within the exercise:

if   belief(pa(T:TIME, person1, A:ATTRIBUTE, B:BODYPART, V:reals),pos)

 and R:reals=1/(T:TIME +1)

then valuation(pa(T:TIME, person1, A:ATTRIBUTE, B:BODYPART, V:reals),c0,R:reals);

if   belief(deviation(T:TIME, person1, A:ATTRIBUTE, B:BODYPART,V:reals), pos)

 and belief(totalmax(A:ATTRIBUTE, B:BODYPART,Y:reals), pos)

 and R1:reals=V:reals/Y:reals

then valuation(pa(T:TIME, person1,A:ATTRIBUTE,B:BODYPART, V:reals), c1, R1:reals);

Note that totalmax(A:ATTRIBUTE,B:BODYPART,Y:reals) defines the maximal value that occurs for A:ATTRIBUTE and B:BODYPART, which gets rating 1, and all other deviations are normalised using this maximal value. For the third criterion mentioned, first it has to be determined for how long a possible advice lasts. This can be done by introducing the representation

pa_duration(D:integers, T:TIME, person1, A:ATTRIBUTE, B:BODYPART, V:reals)

Expressing that for a duration D starting at time T the possible advice is to reduce the deviation by at least V, and using the following knowledge to generate beliefs about this:

if   belief(pa(T:TIME,person1, A:ATTRIBUTE, B:BODYPART, V:reals), pos)

 and belief(minumum_deviation, A:ATTRIBUTE, B:BODYPART, S:reals), pos)

 and V:reals ≥ S:reals

then belief(pa_duration(1, T:TIME, person1, A:ATTRIBUTE, B:BODYPART, V:reals), pos)

if   belief(pa_duration(D:integer, T:TIME, person1, A:ATTRIBUTE, B:BODYPART, W:reals), pos)

 and belief(pa(T:TIME,D:integer, person1, A:ATTRIBUTE, B:BODYPART, V:reals),pos)

 and V:reals ≥ W:reals

 and E:integer = D:integer+1

then belief(pa_duration(E:integer, T:TIME, person1, A:ATTRIBUTE, B:BODYPART, W:reals), pos)

Given this, a valuation of a possible assumption for the third criterion c2 can be determined as follows:

if   belief(pa_duration(D:integer, T:TIME, person1, A:ATTRIBUTE, B:BODYPART, W:reals), pos)

 and belief(maxduration(M:integer), pos)

 and V:reals = D:integer/M:integer

then valuation(pa(T:TIME, person1, A:ATTRIBUTE, B:BODYPART, W:reals), c2, V:reals)

Within Focus Advice Generation for any subset of the set of criteria used, the obtained ratings for possible advice options can be aggregated to obtain one rating for this subset. In this aggregation process weights are applied for the different criteria used.

This is specified for two criteria c0 and c1 in the following knowledge base elements for this component:

if   valuation(pa(T:TIME,person1,A:ATTRIBUTE,B:BODYPART, V:reals),c0,R0:reals)

and valuation(pa(T:TIME,person1,A:ATTRIBUTE,B:BODYPART, V:reals),c1,R1:reals)

and belief(weight(c0, W1:reals), pos)

and belief(weight(c1, W2:reals), pos)

and W1:reals * R0:reals + W2:reals * R1:reals = R2:reals

then aggregated_valuation(pa(T:TIME,person1,A:ATTRIBUTE,B:BODYPART, V:reals), c0, c1, R2:reals);

One possibility is to apply such an aggregation to the set of *all* criteria considered. From the overall aggregated ratings, those above a certain threshold can be selected, using the following:

if   aggregated_valuation(pa(T:TIME, person1, A:ATTRIBUTE, B:BODYPART, V:reals), c0, c1, ..., R2:reals)

and belief(threshold(c0, c1, ..., R1:reals)

and R2:reals > R1:reals

then belief(fa(T:TIME, person1, A:ATTRIBUTE, B:BODYPART, V:reals),pos);

But it is also possible to not aggregate any of the ratings, or only for some proper subsets, and use thresholds in a more differentiated form. For example, for two separate criteria c0 and c1, different thresholds can be used:

if   valuation(pa(T:TIME,person1, A:ATTRIBUTE, B:BODYPART, V:reals), c0, R0:reals)

and valuation(pa(T:TIME,person1, A:ATTRIBUTE, B:BODYPART, V:reals), c1, R1:reals)

and belief(threshold(c0, W0:reals), pos)

and belief(threshold(c1, W1:reals), pos)

and R0:reals > W0:reals

and R1:reals > W1:reals

then belief(fa(T:TIME, person1, A:ATTRIBUTE, B:BODYPART, V:reals), pos);

6.6 Evaluation

This section briefly describes the experiments to evaluate the approach and summarizes some of the results.

Experiments

One male subject participated in this study, who had infrared light emitting diodes applied at fifth metatarsophalangeal joint, calcaneus, lateral malleolus, lateral epicondyle of the femur, greater trochanter and acromion. The subject performed the STS task various times, while sagittal-plane positional data of these anatomical landmarks were collected at 200Hz using an Optotrak (Northern Digital, Waterloo, Ontario) system, and ground reaction forces were measured using a force platform (Kistler 9281B, Kistler Instruments Corp., Amherst, New York). The positional data were used to calculate segment angle time histories and, by numerical differentiation, segment angular velocities. Also, kinematic information and ground reaction forces were combined in an inverse-dynamics analysis (Elftman [13]) to obtain net joint moments.

The actual coaching with a focus advice set
For the proof of principle that the automatic coach could get the subject to make his motion $op(t)$ more similar to the ideal motion $ip(t)$, an advice set had to be specified. According to the literature, the variables in the STS task that have the strongest effect on the peak knee extension moment are initial foot position (Kawagoe, Tajima and Chosa [16]), speed of movement execution (Pai and Rogers [17]) and hip flexion (Doorenbosch, Harlaar, Roebroeck, Lankhorst [11]). Therefore the following focus advice set was used: (1) difference between $op(t)$ and $ip(t)$ in initial angle of the lower legs, normalised for the peak value in $ip(t)$ and weighted by 0.9, (2) difference between $op(t)$ and $ip(t)$ in peak angular velocity of the upper legs, normalized for the peak value in $ip(t)$ and weighted by 0.5, and (3) difference between $op(t)$ and $ip(t)$ in minimal angle of HAT reached during the motion, normalized for the minimum angle of HAT reached in $ip(t)$ and weighted by 0.7. After each trial, the largest of the three elements in the focus advice set was used to give an advice to the subject; this feedback was provided within 15 seconds after completion of the trial, during postprocessing of the experimental data. In the end, the maximum knee joint moment was calculated for each of the STS movements, and in particular it was determined if in the last $op(t)$ this maximum knee joint moment was reduced relative to that in the first $op(t)$.

Results
Figure 6.8, taken from (Aarts et al. [3]) shows an example of how, over a series of six trials, the subject was able to reduce the values in the advice set. The solid black markers indicate the variables for which the focus advice was given by the coach after the different trials. For example, after trial 1 the advice was focused on the peak thigh angular velocity, and after trial 2 on the minimal HAT angle.

Figure 6.9, also taken from (Aarts et al. [3]) shows that the behavioural change shown in Fig. 6.8 was in fact accompanied by a reduction in peak knee extension moment from almost 200 Nm to roughly between 50 and 100 Nm. Note that the peak knee extension moment did not decrease monotonically. One reason for this may be that the ideal pattern and its initial situation were generated using a standard set of parameter values, i.e. without using a subject-specific set of parameter values. Another reason for this may be that focus variables used in this application do not fully determine the peak knee extension moment.

6.7 Discussion

The agent-based ambient system presented in this chapter supports persons in learning specific movement patterns. It serves as a personal coach that observes and analyses a person's movement pattern. The analysis is done by comparing it with an

Fig. 6.8 Focus variables as a function of trial number during an example learning process consisting of 6 STS movements. The solid black markers indicate advice given

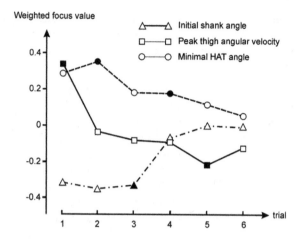

Fig. 6.9 Peak knee extension moment as a function of trial number during an example learning process consisting of 6 STS movements; see also Fig. 6.8

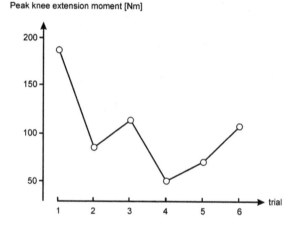

ideal pattern which is generated by optimisation using a computational model for this type of pattern. The analysis is used by the Personal Coach to generate advice to adapt the person's pattern in order to better approximate the ideal pattern. The Personal Coach has been designed using the agent design method DESIRE (Brazier, Jonker and Treur [8]), thereby reusing available generic agent models (Brazier, Jonker and Treur [7]; Bosse, Hoogendoorn, Klein, and Treur [6]).

Based on the agent model designed in the DESIRE environment, an experimental setup was developed. In addition to the DESIRE design environment, this setup makes use of Matlab and Optotrak and the Kistler force plate for the sensoring of body part positions and forces, respectively. Different strategies for focusing were incorporated in different experiments that were conducted, one of which was described in Sec. 6.6. Alternatives for presentation of advice by the Personal Coach were offered in text, in speech (by a supervisor reading the advice generated), or in visualised pictorial form (by means of a simple stick diagram). In these experiments a substantial improvement of the movement pattern in the direction of the ideal pattern was found, which was accompanied by a decrease in the criterion variable, i.e. peak knee extension moment. Further experiments with a larger number of subjects will be needed to draw statistically sound conclusions about the effectiveness of the coach and the way in which this effectiveness depends on specific choices made in focusing and presentation.

Acknowledgments The authors are grateful to Lars Aarts, Kaj Emanuel, and Ingmar de Vries for providing the empirical data discussed in Sec. 6.6.

References

1. Aarts, E., Grotenhuis, F. (2011). Ambient Intelligence 2.0: Towards Synergetic Prosperity. Journal of Ambient Intelligence and Smart Environments 3, 3–11.
2. Aarts, E., Harwig, R., and Schuurmans, M. (2001). Ambient Intelligence. In: P. Denning (ed.), The Invisible Future, McGraw Hill, New York, pp. 235–250.
3. Aarts, L. Emanuel, K., and Vries, I. de (2011). Een hulp bij het opstaan: Project geautomatiseerde coaching (in Dutch). Report, VU University Amsterdam, Faculty of Human Movement Sciences.
4. Bobbert, M.F., Casius, L.J. (2011). Spring-like leg behaviour, musculoskeletal mechanics and control in maximum and submaximum height human hopping. Philos Trans R Soc Lond B Biol Sci. 366, 1516–1529.
5. Bosse, T., Both, F., Gerritsen, C., Hoogendoorn, M., Treur, J., (2012) Methods for Model-Based Reasoning within Agent-Based Ambient Intelligence Applications. Knowledge-Based Systems 27, 190–210.
6. Bosse, T., Hoogendoorn, M., Klein, M.C.A., and Treur, J. (2011). An Ambient Agent Model for Monitoring and Analysing Dynamics of Complex Human Behaviour. Journal of Ambient Intelligence and Smart Environments 3, 283–303.
7. Brazier, F.M.T., Jonker, C.M., and Treur, J. (2000). Compositional Design and Reuse of a Generic Agent Model. Applied Artificial Intelligence 14, 491–538.
8. Brazier, F.M.T., Jonker, C.M., and Treur, J. (2002). Principles of Component-Based Design of Intelligent Agents. Data and Knowledge Engineering 41, 1–28.
9. Casius, L.J., Bobbert, M., van Soest, A.J. (2004). Forward Dynamics of Two-Dimensional Skeletal Models. A Newton-Euler Approach. Journal of applied biomechanics 20, 421–449.
10. De Morree et al. (2006), Inspannigsfysiologie, oefentherapie en training, 158, Bohn Stafleu van Lochum, Houten.
11. Doorenbosch, C.A., Harlaar, J., Roebroeck, M.E., Lankhorst, G.J. (1994). Two strategies of transferring from sit-to-stand: the activation of monoarticular and biarticular muscles. J Biomech. 27, 1299–1307.
12. Ebashi, S., Endo, M. (1968). Calcium ion and muscle contraction. Prog Biophys Mol Biol. 18, 123–83.
13. Elftman, H. (1939). Forces and energy changes in the leg during walking. Am J Physiol. 125, 339–356.
14. Hatze, H. (1977). A myocybernetic control model of skeletal muscle. Biol Cybern. 20, 103–119.
15. Janssen, W.G.M., Bussmann, H.B.J., and Stam, H.J. (2002). Determinants of a sit-to-stand movement: a review. Physical Therapy 82, 866–879.
16. Kawagoe, S., Tajima, N., Chosa, E., et al. (2000). Biomechanical analysis of effects of foot placement with varying chair height on the motion of standing up. J Orthop Sci. 5, 124–133.

17. Pai, Y.C., Rogers, M.W. (1991). Speed variation and resultant joint torques during sit-to-stand. Arch Phys Med Rehabil 72, 881–885.
18. Riva, G., Vatalaro, F., Davide, F., Alcañiz, M. (eds.) (2005). Ambient Intelligence. IOS Press.
19. Sadri, F. (2011). Ambient intelligence, a survey. ACM Computing Surveys 43, 1–66.
20. Treur, J., (2008). On Human Aspects in Ambient Intelligence. In: Proc of the First Intern. Workshop on Human Aspects in Ambient Intelligence. Published in: M. Mühlhäuser, et al. (eds.), Constructing Ambient Intelligence: AmI-07 Workshops Proceedings. Communications in Computer and Information Science (CCIS), vol. 11, Springer Verlag, pp. 262–267.
21. van Soest, A.J., Bobbert, M.F. (1993). The contribution of muscle properties in the control of explosive movements. Biol Cybern. 69, 195–204.
22. van Soest, A.J., Casius, L.J. (2003). The merits of a parallel genetic algorithm in solving hard optimization problems. J Biomech Eng. 125, 141–6.
23. van Soest, A.J., Schwab, A.L., Bobbert, M.F., van Ingen Schenau, G.J. (1993). The influence of the biarticularity of the gastrocnemius muscle on vertical jumping achievement. J Biomech. 26, 1–8.
24. Winter, D.A. (1990). Biomechanics and motor control of human movement, Wiley & Sons edition, New York.
25. Yoshioka, S., Nagano, A., Himeno, R., and Fukashiro, S. (2007). Computation of the kinematics and the minimum peak joint moments of sit-to-stand movements. BioMedical Engineering OnLine 6, 26.

Chapter 7
Using Multiple Self Theory of Planner and Doer as a Virtual Coaching Framework for Changing Lifestyles: The Role of Expert, Motivator and Mentor Coaches

Peter H. M. P. Roelofsma and Sevim Kurt

7.1 Introduction

This chapter will present a framework that aims to be a guide in how to model digital agents in helping people to change their lifestyle, like breaking a sedentary life style and increase the overall level of physical activity. Although breaking of the sedentary lifestyle is used as an example to illustrate the framework, the framework is also applicable for changing life styles that are related to interpersonal dilemma's, like addiction, procrastination, and food-problems.

There is a worldwide acceptance among medical authorities that physical activity constitutes a fundamental element of healthyliving [1]. However, research also demonstrates that more than 70 % of adults fail to meet current physical activity recommendations [2]. In addition, problems related to physical inactivity nowadays are one of the major behavioral risk factors to health in modern society [3].

Physical activity is an essential part of healthy living, although it is in some cases difficult for people to perform. Astrup [4] concludes that currently issues concerning healthy living and physical activity are becoming increasingly prevalent, especially in developed countries. The occurrence of obesity, for example, is increasing rapidly in all age groups in most EU countries and is one of the fastest growing epidemics. He also observes that there is vigorous evidence from cross-sectional and longitudinal studies to support that physical inactivity is one of the risk factors for weight increase and obesity [5]. The conclusion, that people in general and specific target groups in particular have to be more physically active, seems to be a given fact. Focus for new approaches that achieve this is urgently needed.

P. H. M. P. Roelofsma (✉) · S. Kurt
Department of Computer Science, VUA University,
De Boelelaan 1081a, 1081 HV Amsterdam, The Netherlands
e-mail: p.h.m.p.roelofsma@vu.nl

T. Bosse et al. (eds.), *Human Aspects in Ambient Intelligence*,
Atlantis Ambient and Pervasive Intelligence 8, DOI: 10.2991/978-94-6239-018-8_7,
© Atlantis Press and the authors 2013

7.2 Virtual Coaching

Recently there is a growing amount of studies on different kinds of *'serving' digital agents* or virtual agents designed to help people in daily task activities. Research by Lin et al. [6] has confirmed that virtual agents can be effective in several domains: especially in motivating exercise.

Virtual characters or agents act as a new medium to interact with system information [7]. The characters are far ahead in high-quality graphics and make numerous types of interfaces possible. Another benefit is that they can be helpful for a variety of trainings: for example technical trainings (e.g. nurses, medical students, actors, technicians, etc.) and social skills trainings (e.g. practicing your presentation skills, job interview skills, etc.). In addition, the gender, age, race, physical attractiveness, apparel, or even types of a virtual character can be changed simply in a substance of minutes to match the needs at hand [7].

7.3 The Focus of this Document

This document concentrates on increasing physical activity by mediated communication and virtual persuasion. The concept of virtual characters needs more public attention as it can be very useful in several domains, especially in the health domain. Change in physical activity will be explained by persuasive communication performed by a virtual character.

Yet, in most studies, theoretical frameworks regarding the influence of virtual coaching on human behavior are absent. Even today it is still a question how exactly virtual agents influence people and sufficient frameworks are lacking.

As a contrast to this, there are a great deal of theories that aim to explain how people intend and decide to do physical activity. Our approach is to use the field of social science theory that is developed to describe and predict intentions and decisional conflicts about physical activity as a guideline for incorporating virtual coaches.

What follows is a description of several social science theories on physical activity. We start with a description of theoretical frameworks that focus on changing subjects' intention for activity. This description will end with a discussion on how virtual coaches can be introduced to help people change their intentions to break sedentary lifestyles. In particular we will distinguish between using three separate virtual coaching roles: The expert, the motivator and the mentor role.

Next we will focus on theories that describe why people have difficulty to commit to the intentions they have made. These theories deal with the notion of multiple selves and intra personal dilemma's. This ends with a section on how the expert, the motivator and the mentor roles would fit in such multiple self theoretical framework.

Then follows a short section on how using virtual agents can be a way of increasing overall implicit intrinsic motivation to change activity patterns. In particular we discuss that the dimension of gaming and entertainment that virtual coaches can introduce to 'serious' tasks activities like knowledge acquisition and exercise.

Finally, we conclude that the combination of intentional change theory with multiple selves theory is recommended as a framework to guide the use of virtual coaches that help subjects break a sedentary life style and become more physically active.

7.4 Changing Intentions

An example of an intentional change theory is the Theory of Planned Behavior [8]. Ajzen's theory is one of the most dominant and central theories in the social an communication science domain for predicting human behavior. The theory attempts to predict behavior with a focus on human intentions. Intentions are an important aspect of physical activity behavior, it represents the motivational factors that affect behavior and indicates how much effort a person is likely to devote to perform a behavior [9].

Theories that focus on the determinants of intention provide insight to the progression of physical activity. The Theory of Planned Behavior (TPB) is the most widely applied model of the cognitive antecedents of health behaviors [10]. It is also the most extensively studied social cognition theory and it is relevant to both intention and behavior change [11]. Meta-analytic studies have demonstrated significant support for the approach, which accounts for 27 % of the variance in behavior [12].

The predecessor of the TPB is the Theory of Reasoned Action (TRA). The TPB is very similar to the TRA as the TPB is merely an extent of the TRA. The TRA distinguishes two dimensions in a person towards a behavior: *attitude* and *subjective norm*. Attitudes are degrees to which a person has a favorable or unfavorable evaluation of the behavior; subjective norm (also called perceived social pressure) includes questions on whether to perform or not perform behavior. These two dimensions lead to *intention*, and intention is used to predict person's behavior [13].

The TPB adds a third component to this pattern: the *perceived behavioral control*. Perceived behavioral control refers to the person's appraisal of his or her ability to perform a behavior [14] and would also lead to intention. In addition, perceived behavioral control can predict behavior directly (see Fig. 7.1 for a schematic representation of the theory). In sum, the TPB proposes that perceived behavioral control and intention are the most proximal antecedents of action. The TPB has been applied mainly to predict and explain a wide range of behaviors, including health relevant behaviors such as smoking, sexual behavior, exercise and food choice [15–17].

The three dimensions are underpinned by sets of beliefs. For the attitude component these are behavioral beliefs regarding the perceived likelihood that performing the behavior will lead to certain outcomes and the extent to which these outcomes are valued [18]. For the component subjective norms there are normative beliefs focusing on the perceived social pressure from certain referents and the person's motivation to comply with these referents. The last component, perceived behavioral control,

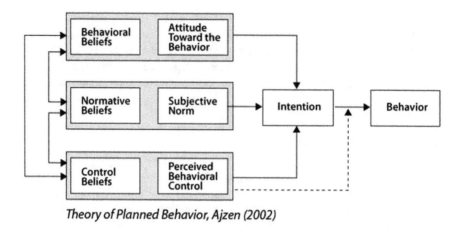

Theory of Planned Behavior, Ajzen (2002)

Fig. 7.1 A model describing the change of intentions

contains beliefs that focus on the presence or absence of obstacles, impediments, resources and opportunities that may influence to the ability to perform the behavior.

As mentioned earlier, the TPB has often been applied in health care; Brickell, Chatzisarantis and Pretty [19] examined the utility of the TPB along with additional constructs in predicting exercise. They divided two kinds of intention: autonomous and controlling intention. The measures for the several aspects were completed during the first phase of data collection. After two and three weeks the behavior of the participants was assessed. The authors concluded that attitude and perceived behavioral control predict intention. They also demonstrated that subjective norm predicts the controlling intention. In addition, they confirmed that intention predicts behavior. The authors conclude their study with the fact that the TPB is a fairly useful model for predicting behavior and that valuable information can be gained when other measures of intention are explored.

Furthermore, the TPB is applied commonly to healthy eating or to physical activity for young people. Yet, nowadays the application is increasingly used with people aged over 65 years. Kelly and Abraham [20] report in their study the behavior of patients older than 65 years amongst healthy eating and physical activity after a theory based promotion intervention. The intervention consisted of a healthy living booklet; it stated persuasive arguments targeting the most proximal cognitive antecedents of behavior specified by the TPB. Cognitions and behavior were measured before the intervention and at a two-week follow up. The authors concluded that the intervention was successful: 34 % of intervention participants set an activity goal, 51 % reported 100 % success in enacting these goals.

Another theoretical approach to human motivation that is receiving attention in the physical activity domain is the Self Determination Theory [21]. This is a theory of human motivation and personality, concerning people's intrinsic growth tendencies and their native psychological needs. Essentially, the SDT proposes that human motivation varies in the extent to which it is *autonomous* (self-determined) or *controlling*. The SDT focuses on the degree to which an individual's behavior is self-motivated and self-determined [22]. The authors identified several needs that appear to be essential for facilitating optimal functioning of the natural propensity for growth and integration, as well as for constructive social development and personal well-being [22]. Here, when behavior is controlled, an external force regulates it. The individual in this instance feels pressured to engage in the behavior.

Based on the distinctions of self-motivation and self-determination, the SDT proposes that three forms of motivation exist; *intrinsic motivation*, which is the most autonomous form of motivation and refers to an inherent tendency possessed by all humans to seek out novelty and challenges, to extend and exercise their capabilities, to explore and to learn. The second one is the *extrinsic motivation*; this can be defined as exercising either to appease an external demand or to attain a reward. The third motivation is *a-motivation*, which, based on the level of autonomy, lying on a continuum ranging from high to low self-determination [23].

In their study, in accordance with the SDT, Edmunds et al. [24] examine the relationship between autonomy support, psychological need satisfaction, motivational regulations and physical activity. Participants of the study were recruited from fitness, community and retail settings. Performance of the three basic psychological needs (competence, autonomy and relatedness) was related to more self-determined motivational regulations. Identified and interjected regulations emerged as positive predictors of strenuous and total exercise behaviors. The findings of this research supported the SDT only in the exercise domain.

According to the theories mentioned above, the ultimate determinants of any behavior are sets of behavioral beliefs concerning consequences and normative beliefs concerning the prescriptions of relevant others. To influence a person's behavior, therefore, it is necessary to change these primary set of beliefs. By producing sufficient change in primary beliefs it should be able to influence the person's attitude toward performing the behavior or his/her subjective norm. Depending on their relative weights, changes in these components should then lead to changes in intention and actual behavior.

As described above, the TPB makes the distinction of three dimensions to predict intention; attitude, subjective norm and perceived behavioral control. Each dimension has its own kind of beliefs. Changing these beliefs will lead to changing the intention to behavior.

7.5 Using Separate Virtual Coaching Roles: The Expert, Motivator and Mentor Role

When virtual agents are used to influence different set of beliefs, the effectiveness of persuasion can be enhanced by using separate agents for each set of beliefs. Each virtual agent then has a separate role in strengthening, changing and updating beliefs.

That is, it would be most efficient to use separate virtual agents for persuasion of attitude, subjective norms, and perceived behavioral norms.

More specifically, an *expert* role can be performed by one virtual agent focusing on attitude beliefs; a *motivator* role can be performed by a virtual agents focusing on beliefs on perceived behavioral control; and a *mentor* role can be performed by a virtual agent focusing on beliefs on subjective norms. This would make for three virtual agents: the expert, the motivator and the mentor.

The assumption is that every digital agent would be 'specialized' in the manipulation of a specific set of beliefs. There are three beliefs sets that need to be manipulated; this means that there will be three digital agents. The digital agents that appertain to the dimensions are: an expert for attitude change, a motivator agent for perceived behavioral control change, and a mentor for subjective norm change.

The reason for this set up is the following: attitude requires an agent that gives general information about the benefits of physical activity. For example the benefits for weight control, examples of performing simple physical activity and so on. Subjective norm requires an agent, which will give examples of other people who do physical activity. Finally, perceived behavioral control requires an agent, which gives information on how to do physical activity.

So when virtual agents are used to influence motivation and activity behavior we suggest to perform studies using more than one agent to influence people. There are a variety of studies regarding the use of virtual agents [25–27]. There is indeed empirical support for the use of separate virtual coaches over using one agent. For example, Baylor [28] examined the question as to whether it is more effective to have one pedagogical agent (mentor) with combined several coaching roles or using separate agents that focus each on one role. The results of her experimental study about learning provide support for the notion of using more virtual agents: separate pedagogical agents representing different roles had a more positive impact on both learning and the perceived value of the agents. She concludes that this provides initial evidence for a pedagogical agent *Split-Persona Effect*; suggesting that separate agents representing different functional roles may be preferable over one agent representing all roles. Linking the empirical findings of Baylor's [29] to intentional theory would imply that every belief set will need its own agent to get manipulated for intention change.

7.6 Dealing with the Problem of Temptation and Intra-Personal Problems

Yet, there are some issue's with the above mentioned theoretical models. Some studies do demonstrate the predicted behavioral changes in physical activity, others do not; often outcomes of the studies contradict each other. One criticism is that the focus on intention is insufficient to explain the paradox that people do not always behave according to their plans and intention. Intentional theories do not take into account issues of temptation and differential weighing of outcomes over time. One theoretical solutions is to combine intentional theories with theories that explain the problem of commitment to intention and temptation. In this way a two stage theory is achieved that would achieve a larger descriptive, predictive and explanatory power.

Multiple Selves Theory (MST) refers to a set of theories that describe the problem of commitment [30, 31]. MST is likely to have an additional value to this research as it explains behavioral differentness as a function of time.

The MST explains the decision-maker process differently than the TPB. In both theories the distinction between a *planner* and a *doer* [32] can be realized. In the case of the TPB the planner indicates the intention. This is certainly reasonable when a person intends a behavior; he or she plans to activate the behavior without actually performing the behavior. The action is not fulfilled yet. The doer on the other hand, represents the behavior; the action is fulfilled, the doer has performed the behavior. The TPB suggests that intention leads to behavior [33]. Intentions actually are important antecedents of behavior, but are not always adequate to produce action. In most of the cases the doer, who activates the behavior, is the dominant actor, and this is the supposition of the MST.

While in the TPB the planner was the decision-maker, in the MTS it is the doer who performance and commits. The multiple self-models have been studied for a long time and different ways [30]. Read and Roelofsma [36] treat this feature as follows. They describe the phenomenon of intrapersonal dilemmas like procrastinations and temptation and explain how the concept of multiple selves explains why people attempt to control their behavior but often fail to do so. Two factors for intrapersonal dilemmas are discussed: the individual actor, that is a bundle of egoistic 'selves', all of which put more weight on their own desires than on the desires of their compatriots (also called personal- or social selves). The second factor is experienced utility; the happiness that we get from what we choose. Other personal selves can add this utility experienced by each personal self, to the experienced utility. After, the total utility from different selves can be compared.

To have intrapersonal decisions, subdivision of individuals is necessary; as a result, they are 'different people' in the same skin. These different people (or selves) have interests that now and then disagree. One of the most widely applied multiple-self models treats the individual as a sequence of selves distributed over time, with each self-taking the baton, as it were, from its predecessor. The wishes and desires of the currently active self receives special status when decisions are being made. Some thought may be given to the desires of future selves; but the natural disposition is to give them little weight. Anslie [34] refers to these selves as successive motivational states, and argues that they arise because of hyperbolic discounting [34, 35].

Read and Roelofsma [36] model the MTS using the hyperbolic discounting referring to two rewards that differ in magnitude and delay (see Fig. 7.2 below for a schematic representation). The rewards consist of *perceived reward from a vice* and *perceived reward from a virtue*. Virtues (increasing physical activity) are alternatives that are good for a person in the *long term*, but often do not give a positive reward in the short term. Vices (sitting on the couch and watching television) on the other hand are alternatives that are satisfying in the *short term*, but may produce dissatisfying

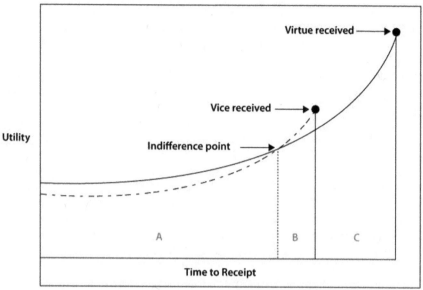

Multiple Selves Theory, Read & Roelofsma (1999)

Fig. 7.2 A schematic illustration of the separate role of the Expert Coach (*A*), Motivator Coach (*B*) and Mentor Coach (*C*)

consequences later. The *utility* depends on the received time, received vice and the received virtue. The reward of the virtue is larger, but the realization comes later. On the other hand, the vice reward comes sooner but is smaller. There is an *indifference point* where the value of the rewards cross. Previous to this point, the virtue is preferred. After the edge, the vice is preferred (see Fig. 7.2 below for the schematic representation).

The crossover point divides the decision maker into three selves: A, B and C. Self A is the self before the crossover point; it has little share in the decision, because the two alternatives are so distant, neither of them are valued very much. When the self A chooses, it will choose the virtue because that has a higher present value. Once the crossover point is passed and self B is present, we can say that the vice is dominant and the consideration of that present now leads the decision maker to prefer it. At last, once the vice has passed, there is a third period in which the decision maker regrets it's impulsive choice or feels relief over it's self-control, that period is named self C.

Similar to the TPB, the doer and planner can be positioned in the MST. The planner is here the self before the crossover point (self A), who wishes to desire the virtue; the self does not activate a behavior yet. The doer on the other hand, is the self who actually makes the decision and that is more often than not the self who prefers the vice; here the doer already took action to realize a behavior. In sum, according to this theory the doer seems to have the last word in actual performance and decision commitment.

Identical to the TPB also by the MST there is the distinction of three dimensions. These three dimensions need three different agents for manipulation. The order of the agents is more diverse than by the TPB. Here, the expert agent will manipulate self A, and the motivator agent can manipulate self B, the mentor agent can manipulate self C. The predictions for the MST can be different than the predictions for the TPB for the reason that by the MST there is a chronological time order that is taken into consideration. Note that self A of the MST can be related to attitude of the TPB; The self B to perceived behavioural control, self C to subjective norms.

7.7 Integration of Intentional Approaches and Multiple Selves Approaches: Modeling the Internal Representation of the Environment

The distinction between a planner and a doer in terms of multiple selves has been made by several authors [37–39] and this has also been linked to models resulting from several research areas like economy, psychology and neuroscience.

In this research the planner and doer activities are often supposed to be located in different location of the human brain. More specifically, the neo-cortical areas are associated with relatively slow thinking processes and more rational thought and decision capacity of the planner. The doer activities are supposed to be associated more in the limbic system areas and are associated with relatively quick thought processes as in intuition or impulsivity. Decision and commitment to action are then seen as a continuous process of conflict resolution in terms of activation and inhibition of these separate brain areas.

Roelofsma [39] integrates these different approaches in terms of what he labels a 'hierarchical internal representation of the environment'. His model consists of several levels of internal representation of the 'here and now'. Each level has autonomous functioning capacity. The levels involve different types of knowledge that describe how the 'here and now' is internally represented. It describes how levels of episodic knowledge make use of procedural and strategic knowledge e.g. for imminent and remote choices. Awareness of the 'here and now' in this model is defined as the currently active parts of the internal representation of the environment.

The internal representation of the environment concerns internalizations of actions and procedures that can be performed or planned in the local environment and in contingent or future contexts. Higher level internalizations may activate or inhibit lower level internalizations. Higher level internalization processes may be deactivated due to resource limitations in terms of attention, effort, and stress resulting in changes in the state of awareness. It can also be due to biological changes like age or cognitive impairment. Each level of representation is associated with different motivational and emotional states.

The model assumes that higher vertebrae organisms are genetically endowed with assimilation processes which internalize action and interaction procedures with the

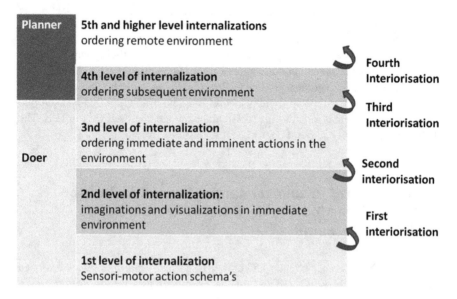

Fig. 7.3 A hierarchal internal representation of the environment

environment. Through interaction with the environment physiological, psychological and social functions are developed through several levels of internal representations. As a result of such *functional interactionism* the organism achieves and maintains a fitness to the environment. In the model each higher level of the internal representation is developed from lower levels through an internationalization process which is described as '*genetic interiorisation*'. This leads to continuous strengthening, tuning, and restructuring of the internal representation of the environment.

Figure 7.3 depicts this modeling of the *hierarchical internal representation of the environment* as an integration of intentional approaches and multiple self approaches. In the figure the planner and doer are represented as different levels of internal representation.

As mentioned the model consists of several levels of internalization. The first level describes basic sensori-motor schema's. These can be formed without much control of the higher levels. Repeated interaction with the environment based on the sensori-motor schemas results in a first order interiorisation and the second level of internalization of the environment.

This level consists of imaginations and visualizations that can be immediately put to action in the local context. The second level of internalization can also be performed without much higher level control when it is sufficiently stabilized.

Through repetition of interaction with the environment using stabilization of the representation in this level is reached and a second order interiorisation process will take place which results in the third level internalization.

Here control and planning of imaginations and visualizations of actions and events in the immediate environment are represented. This level is somewhat more slow than the first and second levels, but still relatively quick to allow planning in the immediate and imminent environment.

In a similarly way a third and higher order interiorisations lead to the fourth and higher levels of internalization of the environment. Higher levels involve meta-cognitive knowledge, e.g. strategic knowledge and evaluative processes needed for future actions or imaginations. Higher level representations also involve higher level emotional states, like feelings of regret, hope or awe. These are also described as hot cognitive processes that are involved in episodic knowledge.

Here planning, higher order evaluation and reflection is represented of different or remote environments. In turn, these are also even more slower processes with allow for more time and control. The virtual coaching framework presented in this chapter addresses each of these levels of internal representation by modeling the provision of specific support to improve the interiosation process as well as the internalization level.

7.8 Virtual Coaches: Entertainment and Gaming

The use of virtual agents has the advantage effect of introducing a element of gaming into activities. Using virtual agents changes a standard serious human performance like a knowledge acquisition task or and exercise into game of playing. This is also referred to as 'serious games': players do not only entertain themselves, they also implicitly learn something from this type of game. These games are promising future educational tools due to the focus of increasing implicit motivation.

Susi et al. [37] wrote a report that discusses some issues concerning serious games. The authors define it as follows: "serious games are (digital) games that are used for purposes other than mere entertainment. These games allow learners to experience situations that are impossible in the real world for reasons of safety, cost, time, etc., but they are also claimed to have positive impacts on the players' development of a number of different skills." In their report, the authors shape three types of serious games: government games, educational games, corporate games and healthcare games. Introducing a gaming element can have direct or indirect positive physiological and psychological effects on the players [40], which is exactly the aim of serious games in health and healthcare.

7.9 Conclusion and Final Remarks

In this document we have introduced a two stage model that provides a guideline for how virtual coaches can be used to help individuals break their sedentary lifestyle. More specifically, following the model we have introduced three separate virtual coaches: The expert, the motivator and the mentor. In the first stage they guide the subject to change intentions when needed with specific instructions and feedback. In the second stage they help the subject to commit to these plans and provide support when they fail. Finally, it is concluded that the use of virtual agents will have an overall enhancement of implicit motivation as a result of the game and entertainment element that it will bring in. We suggest to use the elderly healthy living intervention by Kelly and Abraham [20] as content for the separate virtual coaches and include coach instruction and feedback derived from MST to this content.

References

1. World Health Organization, 1995 in: Edmunds, J., Ntoumanis, N. and Duda, J.L. (2006). Adherence and well-being in overweight and obese patients referred to an exercise on prescription scheme: A self-determination theory perspective. *Psychology of Sport and Exercise*, 8(5), 722–740.
2. Department of Health, 2004, in: M Edmunds, J., Ntoumanis, N. and Duda, J.L. (2006). Adherence and well-being in overweight and obese patients referred to an exercise on prescription scheme: A self-determination theory perspective. *Psychology of Sport and Exercise*, 8(5), 722–740.
3. United States Department of Health and Human Services, 1996 in: Edmunds, J., Ntoumanis, N. and Duda, J.L. (2006). Adherence and well-being in overweight and obese patients referred to an exercise on prescription scheme: A self-determination theory perspective. *Psychology of Sport and Exercise*, 8(5), 722–740.
4. Astrup, A. (2001). Healthy lifestyles in Europe: prevention of obesity and type II diabetes by diet and physical activity. *Public Health Nutrition*: 4(2B), 499–515J. Wm. McGowan, R. Caudano and J. Keyser, *Phys. Rev. Lett.*, 1447 (1976).
5. Astrup, A. (2001). Healthy lifestyles in Europe: prevention of obesity and type II diabetes by diet and physical activity. *Public Health Nutrition*: 4(2B), 499–515M. Lee, *Phys. Rev.***A16**, 109 (1977).
6. Lin, J.J., Mamykina, L., Lindtner, S., Delajoux, G., and Strub, H.B. (2006). Fish'n'Steps: Encouraging Physical Activity with an Interactive Computer Game. UbiComp 2006: Ubiquitous, Computing, Volume 4206/2006.
7. Zanbaka, C., Goolkasian, P. and Hodges, L. (2006). Can a virtual cat persuade you? The role of gender and realism in speaker persuasiveness. Conference on Human Factors in Computing Systems.
8. Ajzen, I. (1991). The Theory of Planned Behavior. *Organizational Behavior and Human Decision Processes*, 50(2), 179–211.Giusti-Suzor, I. F. Schneider and O. Dulieu, in Ref. 14, p. 11.
9. Ajzen, I. (1991). The Theory of Planned Behavior. *Organizational Behavior and Human Decision Processes*, 50(2), 179–211.Giusti-Suzor, in *Atomic Processes in Electron–Ion and Ion–Ion Collisions*, Ed. F. Brouillard (Plenum, New York, 1986), p. 223.
10. Ajzen, I. (2002). Perceived Behavioral Control, Self-Efficacy, Locus of Control, and the Theory of Planned Behavior. *Journal of Applied Social Psychology*, 32(4), 665–683.M. R. Flannery, *Adv. At. Mol. Opt. Phys.*, 117 (1994).
11. Hardeman, W., Johnston, M., Johnston, D., Bonetti, D., Wareham, N., and Kinmonth, A.N. (2002). Application of the Theory of Planned Behaviour in Behaviour Change Interventions: A Systematic Review. *Psychology & Health*, 17(2), 123–158.
12. Armitage C. J. & Conner M. (2001). Efficacy of the Theory of Planned Behaviour: A meta-analytic review. *British Journal of Social Psychology*, 40(4), 471–499.
13. Ajzen, I. & Fishbein, M. (1980). Understanding Attitudes and Predicting Social Behavior. Englewood Cliffs: Prentice Hall; 1980.H. Nakamura, *Annu. Rev. Phys. Chem.*, 299 (1997).

14. Ajzen, I. (1998). Models of human social behavior and their application to health psychology. *Psychology & Health*, 13(4), 735–739.
15. Godin, G. (1993). The theories of reasoned action and planned behavior: Overview of findings, emerging research problems and usefulness for exercise promotion. *Journal of Applied Sport Psychology*, 5, 141–157.
16. Godin, G. & Kok, G. (1996). The theory of planned behavior: A review of its applications to health-related behaviors. *American Journal of Health Promotion*, 11, 87–98.
17. Conner, M & Armitage, C.J. (1998). Extending the Theory of Planned Behavior: A Review and Avenues for Further Research. *Journal of Applied Social Psychology*, 28(15), 1429–1464.
18. Ajzen, I. (1991). The Theory of Planned Behavior. *Organizational Behavior and Human Decision Processes*, 50(2), 179–211.
19. Brickell, T.A., Chatzisarantis, N.L.D. and Pretty, G.M. (2006). Autonomy and Control; Augmenting the Validity of the Theory of Planned Behaviour in Predicting Exercise. *Journal of Health Psychology*, 11(1), 51–63.
20. Kelley, K. & Abraham, C.C. (2004). RCT of a theory-based intervention promoting healthy eating and physical activity amongst out-patients older than 65 years. *Social Science & Medicine*, 59(4), 787–797.
21. Deci, E.L., & Ryan, R.M. (1985). Intrinsic motivation and self-determination in human behavior. New York: Plenum.
22. Ryan, R.M. & Deci, E.L. (2000). Self-Determination Theory and the Facilitation of Intrinsic Motivation, Social Development, and Well-Being. *American Psychologist*, 55(1), 68–78.
23. Deci, E.L., & Ryan, R.M. (1985). Intrinsic motivation and self-determination in human behavior. New York: Plenum.P. Puhl, T. E. Cravens and J. Lindgren, *Astrophys. J.*, 899 (1993).
24. Edmunds, J., Ntoumanis, N. and Duda, J.L. (2006). Adherence and well-being in overweight and obese patients referred to an exercise on prescription scheme: A self-determination theory perspective. *Psychology of Sport and Exercise*, 8(5), 722–740.
25. Zanbaka, C., Goolkasian, P. and Hodges, L. (2006). Can a virtual cat persuade you? The role of gender and realism in speaker persuasiveness. Conference on Human Factors in Computing Systems.
26. Zanbaka, C., Ulinski, A., Goolkasian, P. and Hodges, L.F. (2004). *Effects of Virtual Human Presence on Task Performance*. ICAT.
27. Skalski, P. & Tamborini, R. (2007). The Role of Social Presence in Interactive Agent-Based Persuasion. *Media Psychology*, 10(3), 385–413.
28. Baylor, A.L. (2003). The Impact of Three Pedagogical Agent Roles. Proceedings of Workshop "Embodied Conversational Characters as Individuals" at Autonomous Agents & Multi-Agent Systems (AAMAS), Melbourne, Australia, July, 2003.
29. Baylor, A.L. (2003). The Impact of Three Pedagogical Agent Roles. Proceedings of Workshop "Embodied Conversational Characters as Individuals" at Autonomous Agents & Multi-Agent Systems (AAMAS), Melbourne, Australia, July, 2003Talebpour, C.-Y. Chien and S. L. Chin, *J. Phys.* **B29**, L677 (1996).
30. Elster, J. (1986). The multiple self. Cambridge: Cambridge University Press.
31. Read, D. & Roelofsma, P.H.P.P. (1999). Hard choices and weak wills: the theory of intrapersonal dilemmas. *Philosophical Psychology*, 12(3), 341–356.
32. Thaler, R. & Shefrin, H.M. (1981). An Economic Theory of Self-Control. *The Journal of Political Economy*, 89(2), 392–406.
33. Ajzen, I. (2002). Perceived Behavioral Control, Self-Efficacy, Locus of Control, and the Theory of Planned Behavior. *Journal of Applied Social Psychology*, 32(4), 665–683.
34. Ainslie, G. (1975). Specious reward: A behavioral theory of impulsiveness and impulse control. *Psychological Bulletin*, 82(4), 463–496.
35. Loewenstein, G. & Read, D. (2004). Intertemporal choice.
36. Read, D. & Roelofsma, P.H.M.P. (1999). Hard choices and weak wills: the theory of intrapersonal dilemmas. *Philosophical Psychology*, 12(3), 341–356.
37. Susi, T., Johannesson, M. and Backlund, P. (2007). Serious Games - An Overview. Technical Reports HS-IKI-TR-7-001.

38. D. Kahneman (2012). *Thinking fast and slow*. Penguin Books UK.
39. Roelofsma, P.H.M.P. (2013) *The internal representation of the environment* (manuscript in preparation).
40. Watters, C., Oore, S., Shepherd, M., Abouzied, A., Cox, A., Kellar, M., Kharazzi, H., Liu, F. and Otley, A. (2006). Extending the use of games in health care. *HICSS39*. Hawaii, January 3–9.

Chapter 8
A Network of Sensor and Actuator Agents for Building Automation Systems

Domen Zupančič, Mitja Luštrek and Matjaž Gams

For at least two reasons the energy consumed by heating, ventilation, air-conditioning (HVAC) and domestic hot-water (DHW) systems should be reduced. First, the total amount of energy used by such systems is high: nearly 20 % of the total energy consumed in the USA is accounted by HVAC systems. The second reason is the exploitation of renewable energy sources, which depends on the current time and the weather situation. In short, energy utilization should be improved by effectively managing the available energy. In order to achieve this a network of sensor and actuator agents is proposed for the example of a domestic hot-water heating system that takes into account several aspects, including the presence of occupants. The agent-based schema, combined with the simulator, allows the occupant to choose the most subjectively desirable policy for the DHW control mechanism.

8.1 Introduction

As a result of the depletion of resources and an increasing population, reducing the energy consumed for heating, ventilation and air-conditioning (HVAC) systems, domestic hot-water (DHW) systems and lighting systems is an important research field. For example, in the USA, HVAC systems consume 50 % of the energy in an average building and 20 % of the country's total energy [1]. On the other hand, renewable energy sources are becoming available in the home: residental buildings are able to extract energy from the sun, the wind or even the ground. However the amount of energy produced using renewable energy sources at home is limited and

D. Zupančič (✉) M. Luštrek · M. Gams
Department of Intelligent Systems, Jožef Stefan Institute, Jamova cesta 39,
SI-1000 Ljubljana, Slovenia
e-mail: domen.zupancic@ijs.si

D. Zupančič
Robotina d.o.o., OIC-Hrpelje 38, 6240 Kozina, Slovenia

T. Bosse et al. (eds.), *Human Aspects in Ambient Intelligence*,
Atlantis Ambient and Pervasive Intelligence 8, DOI: 10.2991/978-94-6239-018-8_8,
© Atlantis Press and the authors 2013

depends on the location and the time of the year, which is closely related to the current weather situation. As a result, by improving the algorithms for energy management, energy production and consumption can be regulated more efficiently.

A multi-agent system (MAS) approach to building automation and energy management makes system decentralization possible. Modern buildings contain efficient systems for HVAC, DHW, lighting, safety, entertainment, renewable-energy extraction and others. However, these systems are often managed through a single central system, while small devices such as mobile phones or sensors have enough working power to perform tasks such as usable data processing, data storage and communication. By distributing these tasks among such devices we can benefit in several ways, for example, distributed responsibility, the relaxation of processing power, as well as adding or removing new systems and devices during the system runtime.

This chapter describes how to decentralize a building-automation system (BAS) to a network of sensors and actuators that are able to communicate if and when they are needed for control purposes. In Section 8.2, the related work is surveyed. In Section 8.3, the simulation environment and the simulation model used in our work are presented, while the methods for evaluating the comfort, the price and the energy consumption are also presented. In Section 8.4, the proposed network of sensor and actuator agents used for the control is presented using an example DHW system. Section 8.5 includes the data used for the simulation and the results. The final remarks, conclusions and future work are presented in Section 8.6.

8.2 Related Work

There are many research projects where a MAS was applied to control the systems in buildings. A comparison between the traditional and the agent approach for control systems in buildings was performed by Wagner [2], who argues that the agent approach results in a transparent software structure and dynamic and adaptive application software.

Common wired and wireless technologies, such as ZigBee, Bluetooth and X10, for establishing a network of control devices were critically revised and new Tag4M devices with processing and storage capabilities using the Paxos communication protocol were introduced for a reliable BAS [3]. A wireless network of sensors and actuators was also implemented for a system decentralization of mobile control appliances by Xia et al. [4], while an agent platform for the personalized control of buildings and appliances was analysed by Qiao et al. [5]. The authors of [6, 7] considered an appliance commitment for load scheduling, since the exploitation of limited resources depends on the behavioural parameters of individual appliances. Weather forecasting and energy price were applied to a control system by Escriv-Escriv et al. [8] who showed the potential for further research activities involving control strategies.

Finally, there are complete smart-home projects, starting with the Neural Network House in the 1990s that used neural networks for intelligent control [9]. IHome [10] and MavHome [11] continued with an intelligent multi-agent approach, using several techniques for user-behaviour modelling and predicting their actions. The Gator Tech Smart House [12] is a project for researching pervasive computing methods in a smart building. Research systems often use real data about the weather and occupant preferences for the management of simulated objects, an example being ThinkHome [13].

8.3 System Simulation

The simulation of objects is crucial for the implementation and testing of control algorithms on a large dynamic system representing HVAC, lighting or DHW operation in buildings. It provides the opportunity for a cheap and quick evaluation of a control system's behaviour over a daily, monthly or yearly time period. We implemented the model, representing a DHW system used in a building, where the occupant's activities such as water consumption for a shower, cooking, washing hands affected the system dynamics.

8.3.1 Simulation Environment and Simulation Model

For simulation purposes the EnergyPlus [14] simulator, integrated with BCVTB [15] into the Ptolemy simulation environment, was used. The simulations of the dynamic system were obtained using the EnergyPlus model of a physical system, a weather-data history file and a user-activities history file. The simulation environment is represented in Fig. 8.1. For the preliminary results we used an example model representing a stand-alone electric water heater. It consists of:

- Static construction parameters such as the volume of the water heater or the maximum heating power, which are fixed during the simulation runtime
- Transfer functions expressing the system dynamics, e.g. how the water temperature changes when the heater is on or off
- Input variables, representing the thermostat's set-points, which are enforced by the control system
- Output variables, representing the system states, such as the water temperature or the water consumption during each simulation time step.

During the simulation time step the simulation environment accepts the thermostat set-point and outputs the water temperature in the water heater, the hot-water consumption flow, the energy consumption, the electric energy costs and the occupancy.

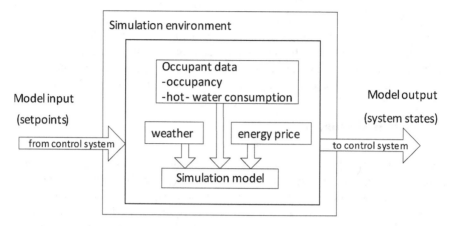

Fig. 8.1 Simulation environment

8.3.2 (Dis)comfort, Energy Consumption and Price

Three measures are used for the evaluation of the system's performance. Firstly, the discomfort t_{missed} is measured by summing the time steps where the occupant uses the hot water for taking a shower, preparing breakfast, preparing dinner and preparing a drink, and the water temperature T_w is below the temperature comfort threshold T_c. Similar notation is commonly used to evaluate the HVAC's operation for comfort [16].

$$t_{missed} = \sum_{t=0}^{n} sign(T_c - T_w(t)) * sign(Q_w(t)), \qquad (8.1)$$

where $Q_w(t)$ is the hot-water consumption volume flow out of the water heater during the consumption. The function $sign(x)$ returns 1 for $x > 0$ and 0 for $x \leq 0$. Secondly, the energy consumption is the aggregated energy consumption rate during the simulation time. Each simulation time step, $E_{consumed}$ increases in accordance with the following equation:

$$E_{consumed} = \sum_{t=0}^{n} P(t) * \Delta t, \qquad (8.2)$$

where $P(t)$ is the power consumed during the simulation time step t and Δt is the duration of the time step. Finally, the price of the electric energy is calculated using the schedule for the high-rate and low-rate tariffs. For each simulation time step the *EnergyCosts* increase in accordance with the following equation:

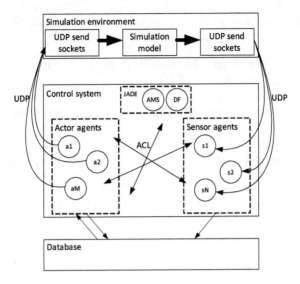

Fig. 8.2 The proposed agent-based control system

$$EnergyCosts = \sum_{t=0}^{n} P(t) * \Delta t * R(t), \tag{8.3}$$

where $R(t)$ is the rate tariff mentioned above.

8.4 Control System

The control system was implemented using agents deployed in the Java Agent Development Environment—JADE [17]. We used two type of agents, i.e., sensor agents and actuator agents, to achieve the simulation of the grid of sensors and actuators as autonomous entities. The control system, including the simulation environment and the communication, is shown in Fig. 8.2.

8.4.1 Sensor Agents

The sensor agents perform two tasks. The first task is to continuously receive the system states from the simulation environment and store the current value. The second task is to wait for messages that are sent by other agents—actuator agents in our example. Such messages include requests for sensor readings, e.g., the actuator agent asks the sensor agent to provide the sensor values for each time the sensor value changes. The sensor agents used in our model are:

- Water-temperature agent, providing data about the water temperature in the water heater
- Occupancy agent, providing data about the occupancy in the building
- Hot-water consumption agent, providing data about the hot-water consumption flow
- Energy-price agent, providing data about the price of the electricity
- Energy-consumption-rate agent, providing data about the energy consumption.

To summarize, each of these agents was used to memorize the state information from the simulation environment and provide this information to the agents that requested the data.

8.4.2 Actuator Agents

Actuator agents are used for changing (setting) the set-point values using the model's input port (see Fig. 8.2), and here algorithms for the control of the dynamic system are implemented. The agent's behaviour represents the control algorithm. Four different behaviours were implemented for the different types of control:

- "On behaviour", where the set-point temperature is set once, and does not change during the simulation
- "Schedule behaviour", where the set-point temperature is changing according to a predefined schedule
- "Schedule and price behaviour", where the set-point temperature is changing according to a predefined schedule and the electric rate tariff. That behaviour differs from the "schedule behaviour" in the extra-high set-point value, which is applied before the high-rate tariff begins
- "Occupancy events behaviour", where the set-point temperature is changing in accordance with the occupancy in the building.

When the actuator agent starts or changes its behaviour, it firstly asks the appropriate sensor agents to provide the requested data by sending a request message to those sensors. If the sensor answers with a confirmation message, then the actuator starts performing the control operation. During the control operation the actuator waits for informing messages from the sensor about the sensor states and changes the set-point value according to the control algorithm. An example of the communication data flow when the actuator agent sets its control behaviour to the "Occupancy events behaviour" is shown in Fig. 8.3.

Fig. 8.3 Communication data flow when the actuator sets its control behaviour to the "Occupancy events behaviour"

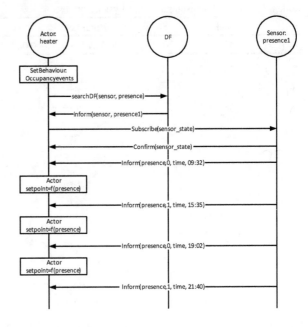

8.4.3 Database

The database is part of the control system architecture that is used to store historic data (sensor states, actuator set-points). Each sensor and actuator agent has its own table in the database to store the state and the set-point values, each with a time stamp. The actuator agents are able to retrieve information from the database. The database part of the control system is created to store the historical data trends of the sensor values and the actuator set-points, which can be retrieved at any time with the purpose of data visualization, analysis, and to be used by advanced algorithms, which will be implemented in future work.

8.5 Results

The simulation was performed using an electric water heater for the DHW in an apartment that was inhabited by one person for the period 25.2.2008–23.3.2008. We chose the electricity tariff rates from the electrical energy provider Elektro Gorenjska,[1] where the high-rate tariff is between 6.00 and 22.00 during working days and low-rate tariff between 22.00 and 6.00 during working days and on Saturdays, Sundays and

---

[1] Web page: http://www.elektro-gorenjska.si/Za-gospodinjstva/Tarifni-casi; Last accessed: 19.6.2012.

Table 8.1 Hot-water consumption flow by activity

	Peak use	Shower	Breakfast	Toilet	Dinner	Drink
Q_w [l/s]	0.345	0.104	0.01725	0.00345	0.01725	0.00345

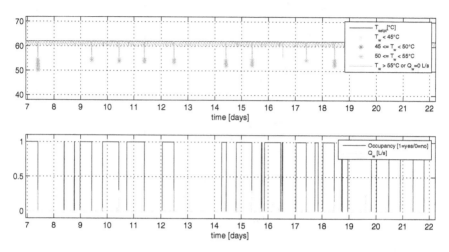

Fig. 8.4 Simulation results for control behaviour—"On": *Top* figure shows set-point temperature for water heater (*blue line*) and water temperature when the water is not consumed or if the water temperature is above the comfort threshold of 55 °C (*green line*) and water temperature when the comfort threshold at 55, 50, 45 °C (*green, brown, red stars* respectively) is not met. *Bottom* figure shows occupancy (*blue line*) and hot-water consumption flow (*red line*)

holidays. The high-rate and low-rate tariffs were 0.07315 and 0.03911 euros/kWh, respectively.

The Kastreen dataset [18] was used in the model for the hot-water consumption and for the building occupancy. The activities *leave house, take shower, go to bed, prepare breakfast, prepare dinner* and *get drink* were converted to a hot-water consumption flow, as listed in Table 8.1. The peak use is the maximum possible hot-water consumption flow.

It should be noted that the hot-water consumption flow is simplified. For example, the consumption of hot water for these activities differs in accordance with the temperature in the water heater. During the consumption flow, hot water is mixed with cold water to achieve the desired temperature. To summarize, the hot-water consumption is lower in comparison to the simulated consumption flow in Table 8.1.

There were three predefined set-point temperatures, i.e., *high* = 62 °C, *low* = 40 °C and *extrahigh* = 70 °C, used for the "schedule behaviour", the "sensing event behaviour" and the "schedule and price behaviour". The simulation results for four different types of control algorithms are shown in Figs. 8.4, 8.5, 8.6, 8.7 and numerically in Table 8.2. For better clarity the results in the figures are only shown for 14 days. Days 12, 13, 19 and 20 represent weekend days. The values in the table marked by (*) represent the best values.

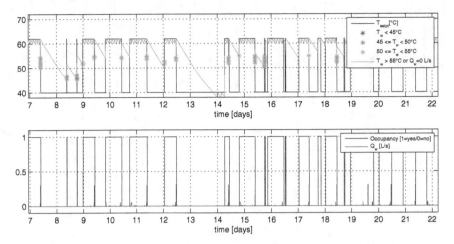

Fig. 8.5 Simulation results for control behaviour— "Occupancy events": *Top* figure shows set-point temperature for water heater (*blue line*) and water temperature when the water is not consumed or if the water temperature is above the comfort threshold of 55 °C (*green line*) and water temperature when the comfort threshold at 55, 50, 45 °C (*green, brown, red star* respectively) is not met. *Bottom* figure shows occupancy (*blue line*) and hot-water consumption flow (*red line*)

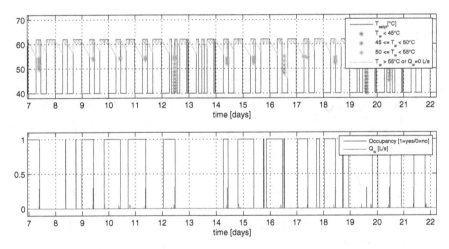

Fig. 8.6 Simulation results for control behaviour— "Schedule": *Top* figure shows set-point temperature for water heater (*blue line*) and water temperature when the water is not consumed or if the water temperature is above the comfort threshold of 55 °C (*green line*) and water temperature when the comfort threshold at 55, 50, 45 °C (*green, brown, red star* respectively) is not met. *Bottom* figure shows occupancy (*blue line*) and hot-water consumption flow (*red line*)

Table 8.2 presents the results of four control behaviours, listed in the first row. The next three rows represent discomfort, where the numbers are the summation of the time steps, i.e., minutes, when the temperature was below the temperature comfort threshold T_c during consumption. For example, $t_{missed} = 112$ min at $T_c = 55$ °C

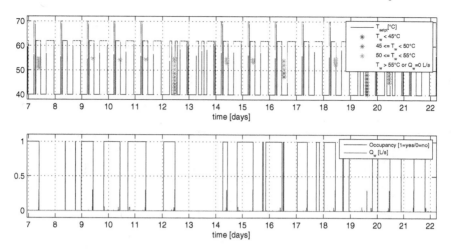

Fig. 8.7 Simulation results for control behaviour— "Schedule and price": *Top* figure shows set-point temperature for water heater (*blue line*) and water temperature when the water is not consumed or if the water temperature is above the comfort threshold of 55 °C (*green line*) and water temperature when the comfort threshold at 55, 50, 45 °C (*green, brown, red star* respectively) is not met. *Bottom* figure shows occupancy (*blue line*) and hot water consumption flow (*red line*)

Table 8.2 Simulation results

	Schedule (behaviour 1)	Schedule and price (behaviour 2)	Occupancy events (behaviour 3)	On (behaviour 4)
t_{missed} [min], $T_c = 45$ °C	8	8	0	0*
t_{missed} [min], $T_c = 50$ °C	22	21	6	0*
t_{missed} [min], $T_c = 55$ °C	112	88	112	85*
$E_{consumed}$ [kWh]	211.789	215.818	208.674*	212.427
$EnergyCosts$ [EUR]	14.13	12.59*	13.12	13.46

means that during the whole simulation time (28 days) there were 112 min when comfort was not achieved. The last two rows show the total energy consumption in kWh and the total energy costs in euros respectively, for each behaviour. For details of the evaluation methods, see Sect. 8.3.2.

8.6 Discussion

Using the given parameters our system computed four characteristic control behaviours or control policies, presented in Table 8.2. It is clear that that behaviour 4 represents the best results in terms of user comfort, but the price for the energy consumed and the electricity costs are higher, compared to behaviour 3. Behaviour 3 is better when the energy consumption is important. If we overlook six minutes in a month when the temperature falls below 50 °C, then this behaviour is better than the others. Behaviour 1 is the worst option. The reason for the poor performance in the case of energy costs and comfort is the poor schedule setting, which was created manually, without the energy costs and the user occupancy being taken into account. Behaviour 2 is an improvement over behaviour 1 in terms of energy costs, but the comfort is not significantly improved, while the energy consumption is increased.

However, it is up to the specific user to decide for any of the four characteristic control behaviours. The task of the system was to compute and present the results to the occupant, so that he/she can make an informed choice. Later, when the occupant's consumption changes, he/she can repeat the simulation if desired.

8.7 Conclusion and Future Work

This chapter presents a system architecture based on the distributed-agent control of a building automation system. The architecture is general and flexible and uses standardized agent communication language (ACL) between the developed sensor and actuator agents. For the actuator agents, several control behaviours were implemented and the results show the potential of a multi-agent approach control. The proposed control system enables a user-behaviour model to be employed for energy-management systems in buildings. The main advantages of the system are:

- A flexible agent-based ambient-intelligence simulation
- Enabling occupants to make informed decisions based on characteristic behaviours of the local DHW system, adapted to each particular user's consumption

Further research should apply the developed control system on a complex simulation model where HVAC system will also be included. Thus, an extension of the agent architecture is necessary, where agents of the higher level (i.e., the management level) have to be developed to combine the top-down approach with the bottom-up approach. Control algorithms based on an analysis of the historical data trends are in development, and for a more reliable evaluation of the improvements a simulation over a longer period of time will be performed.

Acknowledgments Operation part financed by the European Union, European Social Fund. Operation implemented in the framework of the Operational Programme for Human Resources Development for the Period 2007-2013, Priority axis 1: Promoting entrepreneurship and adaptability, Main type of activity 1.1.: Experts and researchers for competitive enterprises.

References

1. L. Prez-Lombard, J. Ortiz, and C. Pout, A review on buildings energy consumption information, *Energy and Buildings.* **40**(3), 394–398, (2008). ISSN 0378–7788. doi:10.1016/j.enbuild.2007.03.007. URL http://www.sciencedirect.com/science/article/pii/S0378778807001016.

2. T. Wagner. An agent-oriented approach to industrial automation systems. In eds. J. Carbonell, J. Siekmann, R. Kowalczyk, J. Mller, H. Tianfield, and R. Unland, *Agent Technologies, Infrastructures, Tools, and Applications for E-Services*, vol. 2592, *Lecture Notes in Computer Science*, pp. 314–328. Springer Berlin / Heidelberg, (2003). ISBN 978-3-540-00742-5.

3. D. Bordencea, H. Valean, S. Folea, and A. Dobircau. Agent based system for home automation, monitoring and security. In *Telecommunications and Signal Processing (TSP), 2011 34th International Conference on*, pp. 165–169 (aug., 2011). doi:10.1109/TSP.2011.6043750.

4. F. Xia, Y.-C. Tian, Y. Li, and Y. Sung, Wireless sensor/actuator network design for mobile control applications, *Sensors*. 7(10), 2157–2173, (2007). ISSN 1424–8220. doi:10.3390/s7102157. URL http://www.mdpi.com/1424-8220/7/10/2157.

5. B. Qiao, K. Liu, and C. Guy. A multi-agent system for building control. In *Proceedings of the IEEE/WIC/ACM international conference on Intelligent Agent Technology*, IAT '06, pp. 653–659, Washington, DC, USA, (2006). IEEE Computer Society. ISBN 0-7695-2748-5. doi:10.1109/IAT.2006.17.

6. G. Conte, G. Morganti, A. M. Perdon, and D. Scaradozzi, Multi-agent system theory for resource management in home automation systems, *DOAJ-Articles*. (2009).

7. P. Du and N. Lu, Appliance commitment for household load scheduling, *Smart Grid, IEEE Transactions on*. 2(2), 411–419 (june, 2011). ISSN 1949–3053. doi:10.1109/TSG.2011.2140344.

8. G. Escriv-Escriv, I. Segura-Heras, and M. Alczar-Ortega, Application of an energy management and control system to assess the potential of different control strategies in hvac systems,*Energy and Buildings*. 42(11), 2258–2267, (2010). ISSN 0378–7788. doi:10.1016/j.enbuild.2010.07.023. URL http://www.sciencedirect.com/science/article/pii/S0378778810002537.

9. M. C. Mozer, The neural network house: An environment hat adapts to its inhabitants, *Proc AAAI Spring Symp Intelligent, Environments*. pp. 110–114, (1998).

10. V. Lesser, M. Atighetchi, B. Benyo, B. Horling, V. L. M. Atighetchi, A. Raja, R. Vincent, P. Xuan, S. X. Zhang, T. Wagner, P. Xuan, and S. X. Zhang. The intelligent home testbed. In *Proceedings of the Autonomy Control Software Workshop*, (1999).

11. D. Cook, M. Youngblood, I. Heierman, E.O., K. Gopalratnam, S. Rao, A. Litvin, and F. Khawaja. Mavhome: an agent-based smart home. In *Pervasive Computing and Communications, 2003. (PerCom 2003). Proceedings of the First IEEE International Conference on*, pp. 521–524 (march, 2003). doi:10.1109/PERCOM.2003.1192783.

12. S. Helal, W. Mann, H. El-Zabadani, J. King, Y. Kaddoura, and E. Jansen, The gator tech smart house: a programmable pervasive space, *Computer*. 38(3), 50–60 (march, 2005). ISSN 0018–9162. doi:10.1109/MC.2005.107.

13. C. Reinisch, M. J. Kofler, F. Iglesias, and W. Kastner, Thinkhome energy efficiency in future smart homes, *EURASIP J. Embedded Syst*. 2011, 1:1–1:18 (Jan., 2011). ISSN 1687–3955. doi:10.1155/2011/104617.

14. D. B. Crawley, C. O. Pedersen, L. K. Lawrie, and F. C. Winkelmann, Energyplus: Energy simulation program, *ASHRAE Journal*. 42, 49–56, (2000).

15. M. Wetter, A modular building controls virtual test bed for the integrations of heterogeneous systems. (2008). URL http://repositories.cdlib.org/lbnl/LBNL-650E.

16. B. Dong and B. Andrews, Sensor-based occupancy behavioral pattern recognition for energy and comfort management in intelligent buildings center for building performance and diagnostics, carnegie mellon university, pittsburgh, *Design*. pp. 1444–1451, (2009).

17. F. Bellifemine, G. Caire, A. Poggi, and G. Rimassa, JADE: A software framework for developing multi-agent applications. Lessons learned, *Information and Software Technology*. 50(1–2), 10–21 (Jan., 2008). ISSN 09505849. doi:10.1016/j.infsof.2007.10.008. URL http://dx.doi.org/10.1016/j.infsof.2007.10.008.

18. T. van Kasteren, A. Noulas, G. Englebienne, and B. Kröse. Accurate activity recognition in a home setting. In *Proceedings of the 10th international conference on Ubiquitous computing*, UbiComp '08, pp. 1–9, New York, NY, USA, (2008). ACM. ISBN 978-1-60558-136-1. doi:10.1145/1409635.1409637. URL http://doi.acm.org/10.1145/1409635.1409637.

Part IV
mHealth Applications

Chapter 9
From Mobile Cognition to Cognitive Mobility: QoS-Aware, Mobile Healthcare Services

Katarzyna Wac and Muhammad Ullah

9.1 Introduction

Advances in the mobile devices, e.g., enriched computation resources, improved storage and wireless communication capabilities and devices' miniaturization, propelled by the need to provide user-centric applications, have accelerated the development of so-called context-aware (CA) systems. After Dey, context is defined as *"any information that can be used to characterize the situation of an entity, where the entity is a person, place, or object that is considered relevant to the interaction between a user and an application, including the user and application themselves"* [1]. This context may include any human aspects that translate to the user's context, e.g., user's health state. In turn, based on the user and application context, the CA systems provide relevant data/information and services to the user, where relevancy depends on the user's task at hand.

For a success of any CA system, it is critical that its user is able to get intuitive and convenient access to the services he needs in a given situation. However, the major challenge lays in a reliable collection of the context data, and service adaptation, especially as the user's context, as well as the needs, changes.

Our vision is that a forthcoming generation of intelligent CA systems collects data using a multitude of diverse ubiquitous sensors embedded in user's devices (e.g., smartphone) and environment, processes this data to learn upon a model of the 'user's world'; his patterns of habits, situations and usual contexts that associate him daily [2]. Necessarily, these CA systems need to collect data and learn new patterns continuously along the user's movements in his spatial-temporal, personal,

K. Wac (✉)
Institute of Services Science, University of Geneva, 1227 Carouge, GE, Switzerland
e-mail: katarzyna.wac@unige.ch

M. Ullah
School of Computing, Blekinge Institute of Technology, 371 79 Karlskrona, Sweden
e-mail: muhammad.ullah@bth.se

T. Bosse et al. (eds.), *Human Aspects in Ambient Intelligence*,
Atlantis Ambient and Pervasive Intelligence 8, DOI: 10.2991/978-94-6239-018-8_9,
© Atlantis Press and the authors 2013

professional, social, intellectual, technological, etc., spaces. As a *pattern* we define a reliable sample of traits, acts, tendencies, or other characteristics of a user or his environment as observable from the sensors. In the CA system, a pattern is then represented as an (ICT) artifact derived from the collected sensor data. The process of the CA system dedicated to continuous learning upon 'user's world' we denote as a *mobile cognition*. Moreover, we envision that based on the learned patterns, the CA system adapts itself proactively and intelligently to the changing contexts to meet changing user's needs. The system adaptation decisions along the users movements are based on the previously acquired data. This proactive adaptation process we denote as a *cognitive mobility*—where adaptation decisions and mobility choices of the user's tasks in his diverse spaces are made based on the learned patterns. Therefore, our vision is that the next generation of CA systems is intelligent and it uses a mobile cognition concept (as a 'knowledge' pane) for its cognitive mobility to successfully satisfy needs of a (mobile) user of its CA services.

We illustrate that vision for a *Quality of Service* (QoS) management case, where the mobile service considers human aspects like the user's health as a context, to which it adapts intelligently its service delivery. The QoS itself is defined as "a collective effect of service performances which determine the degree of satisfaction of a user of the service" [3] (ITU 2008). The QoS management is a mobile service process that aims at assurance that the service's provided QoS meets the user's required QoS [4]. For any interactive mobile service, requiring application data exchange between a mobile user and an (fixed) application server, the service level provided to a user largely depends on the QoS provided by the underlying heterogeneous networking environments supporting the application data exchange. In turn, the QoS provided by these environments depend on the performance of (wireless) access networks available at a given user's context: his location and time, available network providers (e.g. AT&T) and their access technologies (3G, 4G/WLAN). The QoS provided by these environments is unknown for an operational mobile service; it results in 'best-effort' service provisions.

Current QoS management solutions for mobile services [4] result in a large divergence between the anytime-anywhere-anyhow service user's requirements and needs and the actual 'best-effort' here-and-now-service provisions. The question arises on how a mobile service with particular user's QoS requirements can be aware of the QoS provided by diverse networks in a given user's context, and this to facilitate the handover to better network or to make intelligent application's adaptation decisions.

As a solution, we envision a *QoS-information System (QoSIS)* that provides that knowledge to mobile services. On one hand this system facilitates a cognitive mobility process by predicting the QoS along the user's changing context and needs (anytime-anywhere-anyhow) based on the QoS patterns learned from the data accumulated along the past service experiences in different user contexts. On the other hand, QoSIS enables use of a mobile cognition process as it facilitates the QoS management process by providing the service with QoS predictions for QoS of diverse networks in given user's context.

We demonstrate the QoSIS efficiency and effectiveness, enabling intelligent mobile service delivery in the mhealth domain, where the human aspect influencing the service delivery is human health state. Applications in this domain, like remote health telemonitoring and teletreatment [5], pose strict QoS requirements, since a patient can be in an emergency requiring an immediate feedback, e.g., activating his wearable defibrillator [6].

Section 9.2 of this chapter includes work areas related to the context-aware systems at large, while Sect. 9.3 presents work areas related to the service intelligence in mhealth domain. Section 9.4 provides an example user scenario for mobile cognition and cognitive mobility concepts applied in the QoS management of the mhealth application. Section 9.5 presents validation case of mobile cognition concept for an operational health telemonitoring service. Section 9.6 concludes the work presented.

9.2 Related Work Areas

This section presents shortly the related work in the area of context awareness and intelligent QoS-management approaches for mobile computing.

Mobile Cognition and Cognitive Mobility

There is related work on architectures for context-aware systems following the famous vision of Marc Weiser [7]. For example Dey proposed context toolkit [1], Henricksen et al. the PACE middleware [8], similarly Wegdam—AWARENESS [9], Coppola et al.—MoBe [10], Gu et al.—SOCAM [11], and Khedr and Karmouch—the ACAI middleware [12]. All of the proposed architectures follow a layered model of context-aware systems [13]. This model divides a context-aware system into five (or sometimes just three; a condensed view) layers: physical sensors, context data processing, semantic interpretation and data storage, inference and an application layer. None of the architectures include specifically context learning techniques and postulate proactive use of learned user context for an application provision or its management process.

QoS-Management for Mobile Services

Current approaches for QoS-management for mobile services build upon traditional QoS-mechanisms like a session admission, QoS negotiation and reservation schemes [4]. Examples of such work include for example proxy-based proposals of Shah and Nahrstedt [14], Han and Venkatasubramanian [15] or IMS-based approach of Gomez and Sanchez [16]. These mechanisms fail in heterogeneous networking environment, where multiple providers are responsible for providing data communication services (over wireless and wired networks) in application end-to-end paths [17]. With regards to predicting the QoS for a networked application, there exists some research for Internet-based test-beds, where the application is used in a controlled way in controlled networking environments. For example Iannello models delay and losses of Internet paths [18]. Aljadhai and Znati [19] simulate user's mobility and its impact on availability of wireless network to this user. Gao and Wu [20] model server-view delays for web-server clients.

We argue that our approach is novel as we do not propose yet another 'traditional' QoS-management framework, but, based on implementation of mobile cognition and cognitive mobility concepts, we assume proactive application-driven choice of the underlying network and application adaptation aiming at providing its user with the 'best-possible best-effort' service meeting his requirements and needs.

9.3 mhealth: Need for Intelligent QoS-Awareness

This section presents shortly the related work in the area of requirements in mhealth and its intelligent QoS-management approaches.

9.3.1 QoS-Requirements of mhealth Services

mhealth relates to delivery of health monitoring, intervention of treatment services based on the human aspects, embracing the current state of the mobile patient. These services may change their QoS requirements, e.g., real-time versus non real-time, amount of data being sent, depending on the emergency or non-emergency of the user's health state or based on user's context (location, time), as given in the following examples.

Example remote monitoring applications [21] include real-time remote control of infusion pumps that control drug delivery and ventilators that control human's physiological functions, and these require low delays i.e., <3–5 s and low bandwidth ($\ll 1$ kb/s). In this set there exist real-time critical applications for controlling of the human's physiological functions, with delay requirement of <300 ms and continuous low bandwidth of 0–100 kb/s. Maximum acceptable data loss for all these types of applications is $\sim 10^{-6}$. Real-time noncritical applications, relying on audio and video have variable bandwidth requirements i.e., 10 kb/s–1 Mb/s from low (voice) to high (video streaming), require low to moderate delay of 10–250 ms and can tolerate low data loss up to $<10^{-4}$. Office/Medical IT, e.g., web browsing, file sharing, interactive access to patients' records, download of medical images and videos (e.g., X rays, MRI, CT scans) require high bandwidth of ~ 1–10 Mb/s and can tolerate moderate to high delays of <1 s and some data loss rate of $<10^{-2}$. It requires pervasive connectivity and mobility support both inside hospital facilities and outdoors. Reliability for such application is important but not critical.

For a real-time one lead ECG transmission over 3G, having sampling frequency of 360 Hz, block length of 512 samples, with resolution of 11 bits per sample the health monitoring QoS was assessed by a cardiologist. According to him, the maximum value of delay for real-time ECG monitoring, depends on the specific application the monitoring is used for, e.g., in case of real-time interaction between an ambulance and a hospital, no more than 3 s should be allowed while in cases where interaction is not so critical, a slightly longer delay up to 4 s could be tolerated [22].

Additionally when the monitoring buffer runs out of samples, a *stop* is produced in the monitoring process. The cardiologist has also assessed a maximum acceptable number of such stops of data. The results indicate that the acceptable range of 1.7 % stops for monitoring duration of 1 s have been identified, 3.3 % for 2 s, 5.0 % for 3 s and 6.7 % for 4 s in case of 1 stop while in case of 3 stops the range was 5.0 % for 1 s duration, 10.0 % for 2 s and 15.0 % for 3 s duration respectively. Moreover, according to the cardiologist, 3 stops of duration 4 s, 5 stop of duration 2 s or higher and 7 stop of duration 2 s or higher were beyond acceptable thresholds.

Similarly, the total transmission delay of 3 s to an ECG signal being displayed on monitor was reported as tolerable limit for real-time transmission of ECG to the cardiologists in non-emergency tele-cardiology applications using 3G networks achieved through ECG coding approach (block size of 512 samples and the sampling frequency of 360 samples per second). However, it was recommended that the delay limit should not increase much more [23].

An "Electronic Doctor's Bag", which can easily send biological information with multiple high-definition images, enabling like face-to-face communication between the doctor in his clinic and the patient at home was proposed which measures ECG online from the patient home, checks swelling of the patient's foot using smartphone camera and patient's ultrasound echo using ultrasonic device. Image quality with 352×240 resolution, bit rate of $64 \sim 10$ kbps and frame rate of $5 \sim 15$ fps using cellular phone (FOMA) mode was evaluated by three doctors and two nurses and they reported that the transmitted video images for the patient's state were useful in doctor's point of views in non-emergency situations [24].

Kwak et al. [25] have demonstrated two-way, real-time audio and video communication between hospital doctors and emergency medical technicians (EMTs) providing pre-hospital care in real emergency situations using Wireless Broad Band Internet (WIBRO). Their evaluation shows the difference in performance in outdoors, inside building and moving vehicle. In outdoor situation, they observed a Round Trip Time (RTT) of 105 ms, audio-visual delay of <0.3 s with a 5 fps, and RTT of 118 ms and the same audio-visual delay for same frame rate inside the building scenario. In moving vehicle case at speed of 30 km/h, the RTT was 152 ms with audio-visual delay of <0.6 for 4 frame/sec rate and at speed of 70 km/h the RTT was 220 ms with audio-visual delay of <0.8 ms and frame rate of 3 fps. The quality of audio and video transmission, based on the records of the medical control centre staff, was judged to be intermediate, and the transmission of medical information was feasible, even from a vehicle moving at 70 km/h.

Sakamoto et al. [26] investigated the communication performance of the cellular phone (3G) for the ECG telemonitoring in different places with different populations and in the mobility context. The found that W-CDMA communication line of FOMA M1000 cellular phone has enough speed for the ECG telemonitor and it is reliable when using TCP/IP in static fields but have experienced momentary degradation in throughput i.e., below the 12 kbps when using TCP/IP protocol while moving (in the car on the road). In the moving status, the results show that the phone has enough speed when using UDP/IP, on expense of data loss.

Pawar et al. [27] reported the bandwidth and delay requirements of the remote patient health monitoring service are 25 kbps and 500 ms respectively in non-critical situations.

9.3.2 QoS-Awareness of mhealth Services

Given the diversity of requirements for mhealth, there exist papers that address QoS-awareness and service intelligence in mhealth.

To address the adaptation issues for different classes of applications in remote healthcare system a concept of configuration management and context management at software architecture level is presented by Loques and Sztajnberg [28]. Home Health Station (HHS) collects and process physiological, behavioral (e.g., going to the bathroom, sleeping, eating) and environmental data and interprets it in real-time in an example use case for hypertensive patients monitoring. Authors evaluated the system output's confidence using synthetic data generated from exams of real patients, and concluded that the proposed approach performs reliably for hypertensive patients as it relies on averages and considers the vital signs overall history as an possible reason.

To enhance the performance of mhealth system for epileptic patient, an adaptive middleware framework based on dynamic task redistribution is presented by Mei et al. [29]. To support the task redistribution, a computational model to estimate the system QoS performance (i.e., end-to-end delay, availability level and battery lifetime) for a particular task assignment and then to select an optimal assignment has been shown using a graph-based model. This model is based on Task Directed Acyclic Graph (DAGs) that comprises two types of vertices: transmission vertex representing the bio-signal data stream and processing vertex representing the processing of a stream, and the Resource DAG contains two types of vertices, i.e. device vertex representing the available computing device and (communication) channel vertex representing the network connection between devices.

To support the context-aware task redistribution in mhealth system, a middle-ware framework named MADE consisting of four functional phases, i.e. Monitoring, Analysis, Decision and Enforcement has been implemented by Mei et al. [29]. The monitoring phase includes mhealth application registration, device discovery and context discovery/registration. All these information can be represented as the change in the two weighted graphs—task DAG capturing information about the mhealth application and resource DAG capturing information about the mhealth platform. The analysis phase takes these two DAG models as input and runs a task assignment algorithm to determine the optimal assignment with optimal system QoS performance. The decision phase compares the computed optimal assignment with the current system configuration to determine the actual cost of reconfiguration. If the reconfiguration cost can be leveraged by the enhanced performance of the new config-uration, the new assignment plan will be executed. The Enforcement phase controls the mhealth system to adjust its configuration according to the new assignment.

A context-aware and Adaptive QoS-aware (CodaQ) middleware for activity monitoring has been presented by Nourizadeh [30]. The objective of CodaQ is to assess the patient state at any moment using the contextual information. The middleware is comprised of different module to support different layers/services (e.g., Context abstraction, Supervision and QoS, Database, Context processor, Data management, Context router and aggregation, Context provider). The Context Collector, QoS Observer and Context abstraction layer that makes CodaQ as a context-aware and priority-based adaptive QoS middleware where data are given a uniform representation, and their level of abstraction is raised through the use of basic data modeling. The results shown that the total response time of a query in CodaQ system is less than one second (797 ms) where the collection of context data from the sensor network takes 34 % of the total time and the most time-consuming task among the others is the reply time which takes 48 % of total time. The time for context processing takes 14 % and the query generation time is just 4 % of the total response time. CodaQ shown that the automation of home environment by such system, would add an overhead of 273 ms for context collection and 14 % for context processing or 48 % of the total response time which seems to be acceptable as a cost of automation of the context processing and control.

Pawar et al. [31] propose a seamless vertical handover for multi-homed mobile devices incorporating QoS prediction based on context information and demonstrate it in case of remote health monitoring application. The mobile devices perform a handover decision using QoS prediction based on context information i.e., (list of currently available mobile networks, theoretical uplink bandwidth and delay, current state of the network interfaces on the mobile device) combined with the other context information (e.g. location and time) obtained locally from the mobile device. The QoS prediction incorporates different levels of context information including basic information; network type, network name, operator name and authentication, the location dimension which consists of the geographic coordinates of the centre of the network and network radius and QoS characteristics in the time dimension which consist of the predicted bandwidth, delay and the start and end time, and subsequent context changes are for the dynamic selection of and handover to the optimal wireless network based on maximization of bandwidth and minimization of delay requirements for remote monitoring service. The proposed solution results in a higher throughput, lower data loss and lower delay. The work presented in Pawar et al. [31] precedes the research approach called QoSIS, which in details in presented in this chapter.

9.4 Mobile Cognition for Cognitive Mobility: mhealth Scenario

As every Saturday, Sophie visits Westfield-London shopping centre. She is a young Chronic Obstructive Pulmonary Disease (COPD) patient. Her health state (i.e., respiration, heart rate) is continuously monitored from the hospital with use of the

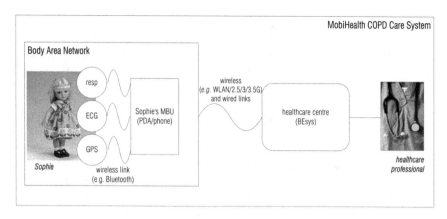

Fig. 9.1 The MobiHealth system for a COPD patient

MobiHealth's COPD Body Area Network (BAN, Fig. 9.1). Her mobile device is the central node of her BAN. QoSIS is deployed on it.

Since Sophie is using the MobiHealth system, she does not have to visit her hospital for check-ups frequently. She feels secure being remotely monitored and being less limited in her active life. In case of exacerbations,[1] help from the hospital is dispatched to her, wherever she is. In the mall, her mobile device always intelligently uses the most suitable wireless access network, as available there, i.e. the network that can send her vital sign data with the least delay to the hospital, but this in a secure manner (i.e., not using any unknown, free-access WLANs and using encrypted channel for all data exchange). Network usage price does not matter, as she has a flat-fee subscription for data communications. The network selection process is completely invisible to her, as it is taken care of by her mobile device and it is based on networks' delays predictions provided by QoSIS. In the mall, her device uses mostly a 3G-HSUPA network of Vodafone-UK, and when it is not available, e.g. inside the big shops, her BAN switches to 3G-UMTS network of T-Mobile (i.e., leveraging the newest multi-homing feature her phone has). In such a way her data is always sent at with the least delay to the hospital. This delay is continuously measured by QoSIS and constitutes a new historical data, upon which QoSIS derives further delay predictions.

It is Saturday afternoon and Sophie is biking to the library in her village. Although she feels good, the BAN warns her of possible exacerbations and triggers an event notification at the healthcare centre. She stops biking and sits on a bench near by. Before she can ask for help, exacerbations start.

At the moment when Sophie's BAN warned her of possible exacerbations, it also collected newest predictions for the QoS provided by different networks available at her geographical location and time. It occurred that the 3G network provided by Vodafone UK is available there, and it has the lowest delays and the highest data

---

[1] Circumstances when a disease or its symptoms become more severe.

rates predicted for the next 30 min, amongst all the other wireless access networks available there. Therefore, the BAN chooses this network and continuously sends all sensor-set data together with Sophie's geographical location information to the healthcare centre. Based on the ECG signals and breathing patterns her doctor sees, he decides to intervene and to send an ambulance to her. When the ambulance reaches Sophie, medical professionals provide her with medical assistance and take her to the hospital. Sophie's doctor prepares an emergency room while he continues monitoring her while she is being transported; her vital signs are automatically displayed for him in the emergency room. During the ride, a prediction of the QoS indicates that the 3G network provided by Vodafone UK will become unavailable, and, given the trajectory of the ambulance, the predictions indicate that the 2.5G network of Orange provides best QoS (i.e., the lowest delays, yet data rates lower than just used 3G network). Just before the ambulance moves out of the 3G network range, the BAN proactively and transparently handovers to the Orange's-2.5G network. When the BAN switches between these different networks, it adapts the data it sends to the healthcare centre. As result, the doctor will not see Sophie's ECG signals when the ambulance moves out of the 3G network coverage and the 2.5G network providing a lower data rates is used. Once Sophie arrives to the hospital, the predictions indicate an availability of low delays, high data rate, secured hospital's WLAN (which Sophie's BAN is authorized to use) and her BAN transparently handovers to this network. As a result, all her vital signs (including ECG) are now automatically displayed in the emergency room.

Throughout the whole Saturday afternoon, Sophie's BAN was continuously collecting QoS-information about the QoS provided (i.e., data delay and data rate) when a given network has been chosen at a given geographical location and time. The collected QoS-information was posted in bursts to the QoSIS, where it serves as a basis for further QoS prediction being provided to mobile service users like Sophie.

9.5 Mobile Cognition: Proof of Concept

In this section we provide a case study of the mobile cognition concept implemented in a health telemonitoring service provided by the MobiHealth system to users like Sophie. We have conducted an extensive feasibility assessment study to prove that efficient (i.e., with regards to the available resources) and effective (i.e., accurate) QoS-predictions can be derived for a mobile health telemonitoring service user.

9.5.1 MobiHealth System and its QoS-Measurements Function

In this section we present the MobiHealth system and the QoS-measurement (i.e., sensory) function of QoSIS, implemented in this system.

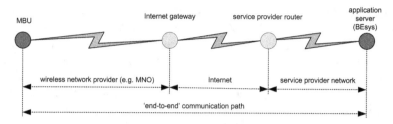

Fig. 9.2 The MobiHealth end-to-end communication path

MobiHealth Architecture

The MobiHealth system is a distributed system for real-time remote monitoring of a mobile patient's health condition [32]. A patient is wearing a BAN, consisting of a sensor-set and a mobile device (e.g. PDA or a phone) called Mobile Base Unit (MBU). The sensor-set is specific for a patient's health condition (e.g. COPD, cardiac) and consists of specialized sensors that monitor patients' vital signs and his/her location sensor (e.g. GPS).

MBU collects and synchronizes the sensor-set data, processes it (e.g. filters) and then sends to a remote application backend-system (BEsys) located in e.g. a health-care centre. The BEsys makes data available in real-time to e.g. medical decision support systems. The BAN uses an intra-BAN communication network (e.g. Bluetooth) for data communication between sensor-set and the MBU, and it uses an extra-BAN communication network (e.g. 2.5G/3G or WLAN) provided by a wireless network provider (e.g. Mobile Network Operator) for data communication between the MBU and the BEsys (Fig. 9.2). The execution of health telemonitoring application is supported by the proprietary TCP/IP based MSP-Interconnect Protocol (MSP-IP) [33]. The MSP-IP and overall system architecture conforms the Jini Surrogate [34].

Application-Level QoS

End-users of health telemonitoring applications are healthcare professionals and their patients (like Sophie). However, only the healthcare professionals can define the QoS requirements posed on the system [35]. These requirements encompass reliable, error- and loss-free vital signs data exchange between the MBU and BEsys at the minimum delay. The use of TCP/IP protocol in combination with the MBU data storage ensures the application data recovery in case of data errors/losses. This chapter focuses on the MobiHealth's minimum data delay requirement; we focus on the extra-BAN communication network delay, heavily contributing to the application delays [36].

The MobiHealth system performance is managed based on the application-level response time defined via a Keep-Alive Round Trip Time (KA-RTT). It is the time it takes for the MBU's control message (called Keep-Alive [33], to be received by the BEsys and returned (without processing) to the MBU. The KA-RTT reflects the delay induced by the underlying networks and the processing delays in the protocol stacks at the MBU and the BEsys. The (wireless) access network uplink (i.e. MBU to the BEsys) and downlink (i.e. BEsys to the MBU) contribute significantly to the KA-RTT. The MobiHealth end-user requirement upon the minimum vital signs data delay translated into the minimum KA-RTT. The MBU's clock is kept synchronized via GPS.

Measurements System Settings

Measurements have been done for health telemonitoring application provided by MobiHealth system to COPD patients (like Sophie), hence measuring patient's respiration rate, and pulse rate, oxygen saturation, plethysmogram as well as user's location. In total 1.5 kbps has been sent continuously by the MBU to the BEsys. For the purpose of this chapter, we have collected KA-RTT traces for one COPD patient living in Geneva (CH), using the application for one month, while following his daily routines. He has spent 69.4 % of the time in two locations: home and office. As the MBU he used Qtek 9090 running Windows Mobile OS. The Qtek used GPRS interface for extra-BAN communication. UniGe provided the WLAN network when the patient was at the University of Geneva and Sunrise mobile network operator provided the 2.5G-GPRS network elsewhere. The BEsys was a high performance server. Both platforms were dedicated for the executed measurements.

KA-RTT-Measurements Function Instrumentation

The KA-RTT values (in milliseconds) were measured every 10 s along the telemonitoring application execution. Moreover, the location, time, network received signal strength indication, remaining battery level and data-rate sent by the MBU to the BEsys (in B/s) have been logged every second.

9.5.2 QoS Predictions Tasks and Experiments

The goal of the feasibility study, as a proof of concept for mobile cognition, is to assess the feasibility of predicting the KA-RTT values based on the data models built from the measurements data. In this section, first we define prediction experiments and secondly, predictions tasks. We also show how the collected measurements data has been represented in features.

Tasks and Experiments Definition

We defined 15 prediction experiments derived from the data or from the following user-scenarios. First is a 'typical' machine learning experiment in which we use 50 % data for training and 50 % for testing (experiment denoted as 50–50 %) [37]. Eight following experiments are defined with respect to amount of historical data available for training, and the prediction time-span, i.e., having 1 day/5 or 7 or 13 or 14 or 23 days of data, we wanted to know if can one predict respectively the 2nd day/the 6th day/the 8th day/the next 13 days/the next 7 days or the 24th day. These experiments are denoted as d:1-1a, d:1-1b, d:1-1c, d:5-1, d:7-1, d:13-13, d:14-7, d:23-1. It can be noticed that we have defined 3 experiments for d:1-1 case; we have randomly selected three different days in a month of available measurements data, and for each day we aimed to predict the KA-RTT value for the next (i.e., the 2nd) day. The next 3 experiments focus on subset of the collected data specific for a given location (home or office) and given wireless access network (denoted as: L1-GPRS, L2-GPRS or L2-WLAN). The 11th experiment uses historical data from 2007 for office location and GPRS network and aims at predicting KA-RTT values for (an arbitrary chosen) month of May in 2008 for same location and network (denoted as L2-GPRS-07/08). The last two experiments use historical data collected for office and home locations for GPRS network and aim at predicting the KA-RTT values for a user's trajectory traversed in between these locations (denoted GPRS:L1->L2, GPRS:L2->L1).

We do not aim to predict a 'raw' KA-RTT numeric value, but its class, and therefore we have defined 9 different classification tasks for KA-RTT. Firstly, we defined classes based on healthcare practitioner's delay requirements posed for a vital sign data delivery. Secondly, we defined tasks based on the KA-RTT numeric values distribution. The first 5 tasks we call 'binary' as they aim to derive if the value of KA-RTT is above or below a pre-defined threshold value: 750, 1000, 1500, 2500 or 3000 ms (tasks denoted as: c1-750, c1-1000, c1-1500, c1-2500 and c1-3000 respectively). The 6th task aims to classify KA-RTT in one of the 4 classes derived from 25th, 50th and 75th percentile of KA-RTT distribution (task denoted as: c2). The last 3 tasks are called 'equal length' classification, as they aim to classify the value of KA-RTT in one of the 5 classes of an equal length between class-boundary values, i.e., a new class is defined each 500, 750 or 1000 ms (tasks denoted as: c3-500, c3-750, c3-1000 respectively).

Collected Data Summary and Data Representation in Features

We have collected in total 1'228'780 KA-RTT measurement seconds for the mobile patient. We distinguish the following features used for KA-RTT classification. Day of a week (DoW) represents a day of the week (1–7; 1 is Monday) and hour (hr) represented as an hour of a day (0–23). We have collected data for one month; if we would collect data for consecutive months and years, the month and year would be candidate features as well. Location (loc) represents the patient's home (1), office (2), shopping centre (3), etc. Network operator (op) represents the wireless network provider and wireless network technology used, where 1 is Sunrise-GPRS and 2 is UniGe-WLAN. Hr, DoW, loc and op are categorical data. The network received signal strength indication (RSSI) at the MBU (sig) has been quantized into four values from 1 (none or a weak signal) to 4 (a maximum signal). Similarly, the MBU remaining battery level (bat) has value from 1 (none or a small fraction of battery left) to 4 (maximum battery level). The variables sig and bat are to be considered as ordinal data with a Likert scale, i.e. one cannot assume the intervals between values are the same but just that the values are ordered [38]. It results the inherent way these values are derived from the MBU OS; they are not measured continuously, but in steps. The health telemonitoring application data-rate (in Bytes/second) sent by the MBU to the BEsys is denoted as MBU-Rout and is a regular numerical value.

Training and Testing Phases

We have used 48 different algorithms (with different complexity parameters) to build suitable models from the measurements data. These algorithms were in the following groups: decision trees, rules, neural networks, support vector machines, k-nearest neighbors or Bayesian networks [37, 39]. Accuracy of classification models built from the measurements data for a given classification task is derived in two phases: learning, called training phase and predictions called testing phase. For a given model, its accuracy is a percentage of correctly classified instances (from 0–100 %). As a training procedure we choose 10 folds cross-validation (CV) executed on a training dataset [38]. In each CV we obtain 10 models for an algorithm. The CV is repeated 10 times to obtain statistically sound training results, i.e., all 100 individual models are then used to estimate mean and variance of accuracy for the given algorithm on the given training dataset. The testing procedure encompasses evaluation of the accuracy of the derived models on the testing dataset. To indicate which models have best accuracy in training (or testing phase) we compare accuracy of each pair of models (hence having 1168 pairs) using non-parametric McNemar statistical significance test. To adjust the p-value level for multiple comparisons, we use the Bonferroni adjustment [37].

9.5.3 Predictions Feasibility Assessment Results

Analyzing the overall results, we conclude that it is feasible to derive accurate KA-RTT predictions in a timely manner having minimal computational and storage resources. The advantage gained from data mining is as follows. All of the results exhibit accuracy of at least 20 % better than a baseline-accuracy derived from a random guess of the KA-RTT class. Figure 9.3 visualizes predicted accuracy values from red (i.e., 0 % accuracy) via orange (i.e., 50 %) to green (i.e., 100 %). Every block in the grid represents an accuracy value for a best model (out of 48 models) for a given task (out of 9 tasks, defined on the x-axis) and experiment (out of 15 experiments, defined on the y-axis). From the figure we conclude that, overall, the most accurate predictions (i.e. of accuracy more than 75 %) are derived for the 'binary' classification tasks (i.e., c1 family) for majority of 15 experiments, with one 'outlier' for experiment d:1-1a and task c1-2500 (accuracy of 50 %). From the figure we conclude that the worst results (i.e. of accuracy as low as 20–40 %) are derived for tasks c2 and c3, with emphasize on the former one. For all 'binary' classification tasks, the algorithms were able to build accurate models predicting if the value of KA-RTT will be below or above the pre-defined threshold value. In the models derived for these tasks, we could see a clear dependency between the features representing location, time and the network used. For tasks c2 and c3, in which we have imposed the classification schema, it was much more difficult for the algorithms to build accurate models predicting the value of KA-RTT being in one of the classes. We presume it is because the imposed classification schema has not been adapted to distribution of any of the features used for the KA-RTT predictions.

We conclude that overall, consistently accurate results have been obtained for experiments where substantial historical data have been used for training (i.e. 7, 13 or 14 days) comparing to a small amount of historical data (i.e., 1 day). For experiments those focus on a subset of the collected data specific for a given location (home or office) and given wireless access network (L1-GPRS, L2-GPRS or L2-WLAN) we observe in general much higher accuracy results across all the tasks, than for the other experiments. Although it is not shown in the Fig. 9.3, from our research we also concluded that decision trees and rules are most suitable algorithms for deriving accurate and timely models for our prediction experiments and tasks. Tree-based data

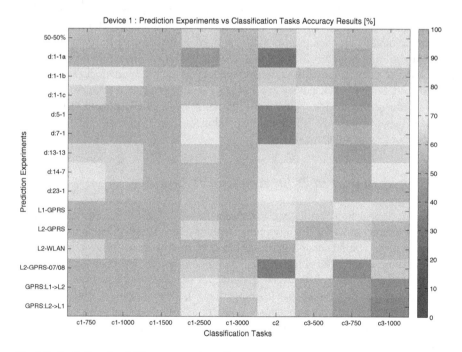

Fig. 9.3 Predictions feasibility assessment results

mining methods, can learn tree-structured dependencies, i.e., our measurements data has been organized in a hierarchical way along the user's location, network provider wireless technology and time features. A similar conclusion has been already reported by Nurmi et al. [40] for research on classifying user's activity based on his location and time. Therefore it is not surprising that when examining the models derived by trees and rules algorithms, we observe that the user location, network provider wireless technology and time were the most predictive features.

The mobile device received signal strength indication and battery fill level were not predictive; it could be because their distributions in our measurements data were very monotonic, i.e., strength indication as well as battery fill level were almost all the time having their maximum value. The training and testing speed of the trees- ad rules-based models is always below 1 s (comparing to hours of training by e.g. neural networks, SVMs) and requires a minimal computational power (less than 10 % of CPU occupancy) and storage (models of on average 20 kB size).

9.5.4 Mobile Cognition: Proof of Concept's Conclusions

Based on the results for a feasibility study for predicting QoS for an operational mhealth service we conclude that such predictions can be derived in a timely and accurate manner. The overall remarks drawn upon the results obtained in this proof of concept study indicate that the previously believed assumption that, it is not feasible to predict QoS provided by a network provider in a 'best-effort' networking environment, may be refuted, at least for case like the studied one. We show that it is feasible and sometimes straightforward to predict an accurately value of a QoS performance measure for a specific mobile application used at given location at given time, while using given wireless network provider and wireless access technology. The prediction accuracy is driven by the amount of available historical data. This proofs our concept of 'mobile cognition'. Therefore, on one hand, we claim that mobile service like the one studied need no longer be condemned to 'best-effort' service provided by the underlying heterogeneous networking environment; an intelligent mobile service can use QoS-predictions to proactively obtain 'best of best-effort' service.

On the other hand, we envision that in order to provide mobile services effectively, i.e., match the changing human aspects and needs and the corresponding user's QoS requirements in the plentiful (4G) networking environments, service providers need to take a necessary step and employ novel technological solutions for the QoS management support. We claim this controversial and non-traditional view on the QoS-management process, as we prove that QoS predictions can be derived for a given service in an accurate and timely manner as a plausible example of such a novel support. To validate it in details, in our research we now proceed with a 'cognitive mobility' proof of the concept for the operational MobiHealth system; besides the simulated scenarios like for Sophie, where the human aspects related to health state, change. Additional, very important variable studied now is battery efficiency [41], different for different types of networks [42].

9.6 Conclusions and Outlook

In this chapter we present concepts of mobile cognition and cognitive mobility, which implementation aims at providing user-centric intelligent applications anywhere-anytime-anyhow—adapting to changing user context and needs, and specifically to the changing human aspects like the user's health state. We have proposed a vision in which a context-aware mobile application learns context patterns along the user movements, thus fulfilling the mobile cognition process, and, based on the learned patterns it then predicts the upcoming context (thus fulfilling the cognitive mobility process). We have demonstrated that vision in an example case of accurate and timely predictions of the QoS provided to a mobile healthcare application operational in heterogeneous networking environments.

Predicting the QoS for mobile application users could help facilitate meeting their requirements and needs 'on the move' anywhere-anytime-anyhow and beyond the 'best-effort' level, as it is done today. We advocate a controversial and non-traditional view on the QoS management for mobile services. Our current work includes detailed validation of the concepts in the MobiHealth system. Besides the 'cognitive mobility' proof of concept, we test an incremental learning upon a new historical data. Moreover, we extend the idea to multiple users collecting and sharing measurements data towards deriving (more) accurate predictions for them, thus enabling provision of services at the ever increased level of intelligence.

Acknowledgments The work of K. Wac is supported by the AAL WayFiS and MyGuardian projects.

References

1. Dey, A., Providing Architectural Support for Context-Aware applications, PhD thesis, Georgia Tech, USA.
2. Kielhofner, G. (2002) A Model of Human Occupation: Theory and Application. Lippincott Williams.
3. ITU-T. (2008) Definitions of terms related to QoS, ITU. E.800.
4. Soldatos, J., *et al.* (2005) On the building blocks of QoS in heterogeneous IP networks. IEEE Comm Surveys & Tutorials, 2005. 7(1): p. 69–88.
5. Tachakra, S. *et al.* (2003) Mobile e-Health: the Unwired Evolution of Telemedicine. Telemedicine Journal & eHealth, 9(3): 247–57.
6. Schott, R. (2005) Wearable defibrillator. J of Cardiovascular Nursing, 2005.
7. Weiser, M. (1991) The computer for the 21st century, Scientific American, 265(3), pp. 94–104.
8. Henricksen, K., *et al.* (2005) Middleware for Distributed Context-Aware Systems. OTM. Springer Berlin.

9. Wegdam, M. (2005) AWARENESS: A project on Context AWARE mobile NEtworks and ServiceS. Mobile & Wireless Comm Summit. 2005.
10. Coppola, P., *et al.* (2005) Mobe: A framework for context-aware mobile applications. CAPS.
11. Gu, T., H.Pung, D. Zhang (2005) A service-oriented middleware for building context-aware services. J Net & Comp App. 28(1):p.1–18.
12. Khedr, M., A. Karmouch (2008) ACAI: Agent-Based Context-aware Infrastructure for Spontaneous Applications. J of Net & Com A., 2008, 28(1).
13. Ailisto, H., *et al.* (2002) Structuring Context Aware Applications: Five-Layer Model and Example Case. Ubicomp, Sweden.
14. Shah, S. and K. Nahrstedt (2005) Guaranteeing Throughput for Real-Time Traffic in Multi-hop IEEE 802.11 Wireless Networks, IEEE MilCom, 2005.
15. Han, Q. and N. Venkatasubramanian (2006) Information Collection Services for QoS-aware Mobile Applications. IEEE TMC. 5(5).
16. Gomez, G. and R. Sanchez (2005) End-to-End Quality of Service over Cellular Networks, Wiley Publishers.
17. Chalmers, D. and M. Sloman (1999) A survey of QoS in mobile computing environments. IEEE Comm Surveys, 2(2).
18. Iannello, G. *et al.* (2005) End-to-End Packet-Channel Bayesian Model applied to Heterogeneous Wireless Networks. IEEE Globecom.
19. Aljadhai, A. and T.F. Znati (2001) Predictive mobility support for QoS provisioning in mobile wireless environments. IEEE JSAC. 19(10).
20. Gao, Z., & Wu, G. (2005) Combining QoS-based service selection with performance prediction. ICEBE.
21. A. Soomro and D. Cavalcanti (2007) Opportunities and challenges in using WPAN and WLAN technologies in medical environments, IEEE COMMAG, 45 (2): 114–122.
22. A. Alesanco and J. Garcia, (2010) Clinical assessment of wireless ECG transmission in real-time cardiac tele-monitoring, IEEE Trans. Inf. Technol. Biomed., 14(5), 1144–1152.
23. A. Alesanco, J. Garcia, and R. S. H. Istepanian (2006) Performance Study of Real-Time ECG Transmission in Wireless Networks for Telecardiology Applications. IEEE ITAB.
24. M. Yoshizawa, *et al.* (2010) A mobile communications system for home-visit medical services: The Electronic Doctor's Bag, IEEE EMBC 2010, pp. 5496–5499.
25. Kwak M.J., et al. (2009) Real-time medical control using a wireless audio-video transmission device in a pre-hospital emergency service in Korea. J Telemed Telecare, 15(1): 404–8.
26. Sakamoto T., Hui W., Daming W. (2006) Performance evaluation of 12-lead ECG telemonitor utilizing 3G cellular phone, IEEE ICC 2006, p. 83–87
27. Pawar, P., *et al.* (2008) Performance evaluation of the context-aware handover mechanism for the nomadic mobile services in remote patient monitoring, Elsevier Computer Comm., 2008.
28. Loques, O. and Sztajnberg, A. (2010) Adaptation issues in software architectures of remote health care systems, Workshop on Software Engineering in Health Care.
29. H. Mei, *et al.* (2008) Enhancing the performance of mobile healthcare systems based on task-redistribution, INFOCOM Workshops, pp. 1–6.
30. Nourizadeh, S., Song, Y.Q., Thomesse, J.P., (2011) CodaQ: A Context-Aware and Adaptive QoS-Aware Middleware for Activity Monitoring. (2011) Toward Useful Services for Elderly and People with Disabilities. ICOST, pp. 96–103.
31. Pawar, P. *et al.* (2009) Context-aware computing support for network-assisted seamless vertical handover in remote patient monitoring. AINA 2009, pp. 351–358.
32. van Halteren, A., *et al.*, (2004) Mobile Patient Monitoring: The MobiHealth System. J on Inf Technology in Healthcare, 2(5): p. 365–373.
33. Pawar, P., *et al.* (2007) Context-Aware Middleware Support for the Nomadic Mobile Services on Multihomed Handheld Mobile Devices. IEEE ISCC 2007.
34. SUN, (2001) The Jini™ Technology Surrogate Architecture. 2001, SUN Inc.
35. Broens, T., *et al.* (2007) Determinants for successful telemedicine implementations. J for Telemedicine and Telecare, 13(6): p. 303–9.

36. Bults, R., *et al.* (2005) Goodput Analysis of 3G wireless networks supporting m-health services. IEEE ConTEL.
37. Witten, I., and Frank, E. (2005) Data Mining: Morgan Kaufmann, 2005.
38. DeVellis, F. (2003) Scale development: theory and applications: SAGE.
39. Alpaydin, E. (2004) Introduction to machine learning: MIT press.
40. Nurmi, P., Hassinen, M., & Lee, K. (2007) Comparative Analysis of Personalization Techniques for a Mobile Application. AINAW.
41. Ickin, S., *et al.* (2012) Factors Influencing Quality of Experience of Commonly-Used Mobile Applications. IEEE COMMAG, 50(4): 48–56.
42. K.Wac, *et al.*, (2009) Power- and Delay-Awareness of Health Telemonitoring Services: the MobiHealth System Case Study, IEEE JSAC, 27(4): 525–536.

Chapter 10
Mobile Phone Tools with Ambient Intelligence for the Management of Life-Threatening Allergies

Luis U. Hernandez-Munoz and Sandra I. Woolley

This chapter describes the unmet needs of people with anaphylactic allergies and considers how pervasive technologies and ambient intelligence might support them in allergy management tasks. A working prototype solution, PervaLaxis Touchscreen, is presented which provides allergy management tools on a mobile phone and communicates with a wireless sensor to detect adrenaline injections. The results of usability testing are presented and demonstrate potential for mobile phone tools with ambient intelligence to provide useful and usable functionality to supplement the traditional system of training and education provided for allergy management. Test participants reported PervaLaxis Touchscreen tools, such as adrenaline injectors expiry date list, emergency support button and adrenaline injection sensing, as useful and stated the information and functions as more accessible by being integrated in the mobile phone.

10.1 Introduction

In recent years pervasive computing and ambient intelligence have been applied to various aspects of healthcare, particularly assisted living and applications supporting people managing chronic medical conditions such as diabetes and cardiovascular disease. As yet, however, there has been little application to allergy management though people with allergies, and in particular people with severe life-threatening anaphylactic allergies, might significantly benefit from the technology both in everyday life and in the event of an allergic reaction.

L. U. Hernandez-Munoz (✉) · S. I. Woolley
School of Electronic, Electrical and Computer Engineering, University of Birmingham, Birmingham B15 2TT, UK
e-mail: LXH615@bham.ac.uk

S. I. Woolley
e-mail: S.I.Woolley@bham.ac.uk

T. Bosse et al. (eds.), *Human Aspects in Ambient Intelligence*,
Atlantis Ambient and Pervasive Intelligence 8, DOI: 10.2991/978-94-6239-018-8_10,
© Atlantis Press and the authors 2013

Using a human-centered design approach we designed and tested a mobile phone and wireless sensing system called PervaLaxis Touchscreen comprising a set of tools to support people managing anaphylactic allergies. User requirements were established by consultations with anaphylactic people, carers of anaphylactic children, healthcare professionals, and attendance at training sessions for patients and a medical forum for clinical experts. These requirements informed the design of a pilot prototype [1], the user testing feedback of which informed the design of PervaLaxis Touchscreen.

This chapter is structured as follows: Sections 10.1 10.2 10.3 explain what anaphylaxis is and how its management might be supported. Section 10.2 considers the users and user requirements. Section 10.3 describes PervaLaxis Touchscreen and Sects. 10.4 and 10.5 outline the evaluation methodology and usability results. Finally, Sect. 10.6 presents conclusions and directions for further work.

10.1.1 Anaphylactic Allergies

"Anaphylaxis is a serious allergic reaction that is rapid in onset and may cause death" [2]. Reactions may occur rapidly after contact, ingestion or inhalation of an allergen which may be a food, a wasp or bee sting, or a substance such as latex or a prescription drug. Reactions to allergens can also be delayed and can occur several hours after exposure.

In allergic people, allergens cause an immunological reaction in the body, which releases chemical substances (e.g., histamine) that produce the symptoms of an allergic reaction. For example, itching of the eyes, swelling of the throat and mouth, difficulty in swallowing or speaking, shortness of breath, alterations in heart rate, a drop in blood pressure or loss of consciousness [3, 4]. In people with anaphylaxis, allergic symptoms can be so severe that they can cause death.

The incidence of anaphylaxis is increasing. Children and adolescents are the most commonly affected. The Anaphylaxis Campaign [4] estimates that 1 in 52 children in the UK is anaphylactic. The World Allergic Organization [5] reports that approximately 29,000 food triggered anaphylactic events occur each year in the United States. The prevalence and the increasing rate of occurrence mean that anaphylaxis could be considered epidemic [6].

The first-line treatment for a severe anaphylactic reaction is the immediate administration of adrenaline given by an adrenaline injector into the outer thigh. Anaphylactic people and their carers typically carry one or more such injectors and also a mobile phone to call emergency services and alert family or friends in the event of a reaction. Since reactions might be provoked by inhalation, ingestion or skin contact with minute amounts of an allergen, it is important that people at risk of anaphylactic reactions learn how to avoid contact with their allergens and are aware of contamination risks. For example, ensuring food has not been cut with a knife that has been in contact with an allergen. Not surprisingly, anaphylaxis has implications not just for the individual affected but also for their family and friends. For example, "invitations to dinner parties and social gatherings become a source of embarrassment and anxiety rather than enjoyment. A simple trip to the supermarket can become a lengthy series of food label examinations and a family trip abroad, if even considered, a delicate military operation" [7].

10.1.2 *Unmet Needs of People with Anaphylaxis*

Following the onset of allergic symptoms, or after a first anaphylactic attack, patients typically meet with a family doctor or clinician, who may make a referral for diagnosis and advice on managing their allergies and preventing reactions. Patients should then be provided with adrenaline injectors and trained in their use. The injectors are packaged with patient information leaflets showing how they are used. Further information documents may be provided to the patients which they may supplement with, for example, on-line resources of allergy groups such as the Anaphylaxis Campaign [4]. However, after initial medical advice there may be little further reinforcement or support of the necessary on-going learning and management processes beyond the documents available to the patient. We refer to this conventional style of learning, training and support as the "*traditional system*".

Unfortunately, the training and information provided to patients and carers can be delayed and incomplete [8], with the result that many fail to use adrenaline injectors correctly and do not have a system of continuous practice [9]. This results in a lack of preparedness which means they may fail to have adrenaline injectors available at the time of a reaction, they may not have an emergency action plan (a summary of emergency actions with useful information and a list of emergency contacts) or they may fail to follow it. Common errors observed in practice include a delay in administering adrenaline or using the injector incorrectly, carrying out unintentional injections (for example, caused by holding the injector the wrong way up and injecting the holder's thumb), failing to hold the injector in place for the required 10 s and failing to immediately call emergency services [10, 11].

There is a global lack of specialists and services, and a need for improved patient care, training and expertise in this area [12]. Similarly, there is a lack of training for nurses and people who care for those with anaphylaxis [13]. It is unsurprising then that the majority of families do not feel confident about allergen avoidance and adrenaline injector use, and feel they lack information and support [8].

10.1.3 *Pervasive and Ambient Intelligence for Healthcare*

Mobile systems using pervasive technology and ambient intelligence may provide an opportunity to help improve healthcare services, decrease medical costs and provide access to healthcare for greater numbers of people [14]. Smartphones and tablets are now everyday items in the lives of millions of people and the range of uses and applications have significantly increased [15, 16]. Although there are challenges associated with aspects of usability, data privacy and security, network bandwidth and power efficiency [17], progress has been made in the technical challenges associated with processing speed, interface design and storage [18].

There are now many commercial and freeware health and wellbeing apps available for mobile users to download. These tend to be simple implementations without formal evaluation. For example, CardioTrainer [19], an activity tracker for runners which uses Google maps and the mobile phone's built-in GPS; Instant Heart Rate [20], a pulse meter using the mobile phone's light and built-in camera to detect capillary changes in the finger; eDiabetes [21] and Handy Logs Sugar [22] which store glucose, blood pressure and cholesterol readings for diabetes management; Diet & Food Tracker [23] which tracks calories and weight; Medlife [24], a medical record application; and Mobile Coach [25], an application which monitors weight, blood pressure and body fat and makes dietary recommendations.

Mobile healthcare prototypes reported in the literature include various systems for the management of chronic conditions such as diabetes [26–28], cardio-vascular disease [29], rehabilitation [30], and activity monitoring for stroke patients [31]. Relatively few research efforts or mobile apps relate to allergy management [32]. Smart Food [33] was a PDA design reported in the literature for allergy users to scan barcodes and identify product ingredients. ScanAvert [34] is a commercial mobile phone app that scans product ingredients and checks them against a user list of allergens. It requires a subscription service. A drug checker [35] is also reported in the literature for checking and communicating prescription drug ingredients with the aim of reducing adverse reactions. Simple but useful allergy-related mobile phone applications include an app for USA users to receive news about allergies and a map of USA pollen levels [36] and Allergy Free Passport [37] to help select restaurants and personalize eating choices. Although there have been positive attitudes towards the use of these systems, there are remaining questions regarding usability, future adoption and clinical benefit [38].

10.2 The Users and User Requirements

The effective management of anaphylaxis in everyday life usually requires cooperation between the allergic person and supporting people, for example, from carers, family and friends.

The allergic person (depending on age) is responsible for allergy management tasks such as managing medications, avoiding allergens, and educating and training others.

Supporting people may be carers (or caregivers), trained supporters and untrained supporters. Their level of responsibility may vary. For example:

Carers such as family members or close friends are more likely to be trained to support emergency and everyday life activities and to have some responsibility for care and allergy expertise. For example, providing help to avoid allergens, manage medications, follow an emergency action plan and, where appropriate, encouraging independence. *Trained supporters* such as school nurses and teachers, first aiders, friends and co-workers, are examples of the people who would be familiar with the emergency action plan and trained to support the person in an emergency, for example, trained in adrenaline injection. *Untrained supporters*, such as classmates or colleagues, may be familiar with the person's allergic condition but not explicitly trained. These people may be in attendance in an emergency and might, for example, recognize a possible reaction event and understand the need to summon help quickly.

10.2.1 User Requirements in Everyday Life

User requirements were established by consultations with anaphylactic people, carers of anaphylactic children and healthcare professionals, and attendance at training sessions for patients and a medical forum for clinical experts. These requirements informed the design of a pilot prototype [1], the user testing feedback of which informed the design of PervaLaxis Touchscreen.

Figure 10.1 illustrates the everyday use cases identified: information about anaphylaxis, adrenaline injector management to help ensure all adrenaline injectors are in date and not expired, and adrenaline injection training.

10.2.2 User Requirements in the Context of an Emergency

Users expressed a strong interest in support for emergencies that could help people see how to give an injection of adrenaline and provide functionality to sense

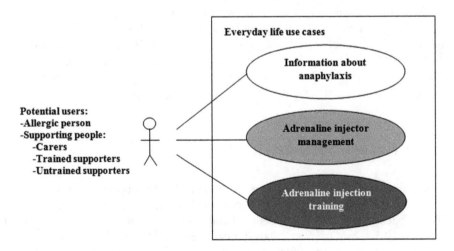

Fig. 10.1 Use cases aimed to support everyday life tasks

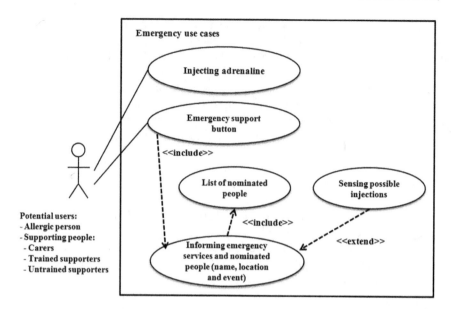

Fig. 10.2 Use cases for emergency support

possible injections and send automatic SMS messages to emergency services and to nominated people. Emergency messaging services that support mobile phone SMS communication are emerging, for example, there is Emergency-SMS in the UK [39] allowing deaf and speech-impaired people, to register mobile phones from which they can send SMS messages to emergency services. A text-to-911 service in the USA is anticipated for 2014 [40].

Users wanted the messages to communicate emergency events and possible injections. They also wanted to include in the messages useful information such as name, location and the event (e.g., "possible use of adrenaline injector") and wanted a simple, visible "emergency support button" to activate these functions. Figure 10.2 shows the use cases associated with emergency use: injecting adrenaline, informing emergency services and nominated people, and sensing possible injections.

10.3 PervaLaxis Touchscreen

The user requirements were implemented in PervaLaxis Touchscreen: a working prototype system comprising a set of tools implemented on an HTC Diamond 2 Smartphone running Windows Mobile 6.1 and a wireless motion sensing unit.

Figure 10.3 shows the PervaLaxis Touchscreen Smartphone and an adrenaline injector mounted on the wireless accelerometer unit containing a SparkFun Bluetooth® Wireless 3D Tilt Sensing unit, battery and an LM7805 voltage

Fig. 10.3 a PervaLaxis touchscreen smartphone device;
b Adrenaline injector with a
3D Bluetooth accelerometer;
c Pen size comparison

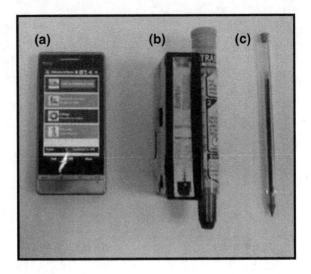

regulator. The unit was configured to sample X, Y and Z channels at 10 Hz. Empirical
thresholding limits were used to detect possible injections. The tools were developed
using Visual Studio 2008, C#.

10.3.1 Tools Implemented in Pervalaxis Touchscreen

Table 10.1 summarizes the tools implemented in Pervalaxis Touchscreen, as defined
by the user requirements in the context of everyday life and emergency and shown
in the use cases in Figs. 10.1 and 10.2, respectively.

Figure 10.4 shows screenshots of PervaLaxis Touchscreen user interface.
Figure 10.4a depicts the welcome screen with the emergency support button.
Figure 10.4b shows the injector list tool to manage adrenaline injector expiry dates
and provide reminders for renewal. Figure 10.4c illustrates the information tool with
videos to demonstrate injections and explain about anaphylaxis. Figure 10.4d shows
an injector trainer screenshot, which was designed to provide a visual demonstration
of the steps required in an adrenaline injection. It was also designed to help users
practice injections by providing feedback on the force applied to the injector trainer
device.

Figure 10.5a illustrates how the accelerometer sensor unit was mounted on an
adrenaline injector trainer. A trainer is a needle-free injector produced by manufac-
turers to help people practice injections. Figure 10.5c shows an example of a received
signal. Acceleration data were analyzed with a simple thresholding algorithm.

Table 10.1 Tools implemented in PervaLaxis touchscreen

Context and user	User requirements	Use cases achieved	Tool implemented in PervaLaxis	Potential benefit
	Manage the expiry dates of adrenaline injectors	Adrenaline injector management	Injector expiry date list	The user can check and modify a list of adrenaline injectors expiry dates
Everyday life	Keep injectors in-date at all the times			
Allergic person/supporting people	Training to use adrenaline injectors	Adrenaline injection training	Injector trainer	It provides a list of injection instructions and provides feedback on sensed injection motion
Everyday life and Emergency	Create an emergency plan. Inform emergency services and carers about an emergency event	List of nominated people	Contact numbers (within settings)	The user can modify her/his contact and emergency numbers list for emergencies
Allergic person/supporting people	Get informed about anaphylaxis facts	-Information about anaphylaxis	Information (Videos)	It informs the user about anaphylaxis and how to inject adrenaline
	Support continuous learning and training about how to detect symptoms, how to avoid allergens, how to avoid contamination and cross contamination	-Injecting adrenaline		

Table 10.1 (continued)

Context and user	User requirements	Use cases achieved	Tool implemented in PervaLaxis	Potential benefit
Emergency	Inform emergency services and carers about an emergency event.	- Emergency support button.	Emergency support button	The user can send SMS messages to emergency services and carer automatically after pressing the emergency button. Name, location and event are embedded in the messages
Allergic person/supporting people		- Informing emergency services and nominated people (name, location and event) - Sensing possible injections		

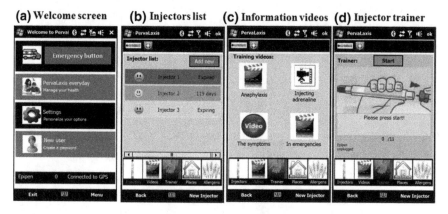

Fig. 10.4 Screenshots of PervaLaxis Touchscreen user interface

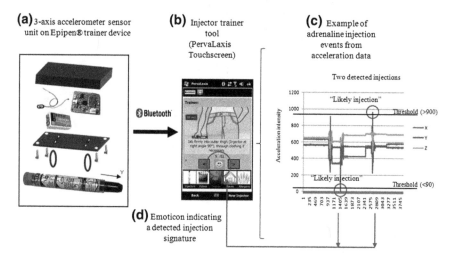

Fig. 10.5 Ambient Intelligence mechanism used to detect adrenaline injection events through an injector trainer tool and a sensor mounted on an Epipen® trainer device

10.4 Study Methodology

The aim of the study was broadly to investigate the potential of wireless pervasive technology, in the form of a Smartphone and accelerometer, to provide usable support for anaphylaxis management. Clinical trial testing normally requires preclinical investigation prior to phase 1 testing, i.e., testing with healthy volunteers. As a new application of technology to anaphylaxis management, the research underlying this study was aimed at producing preclinical testing results that might usefully inform phase 1 and, subsequently, phase 2 testing, i.e., testing on real patients. Of specific interest to the pretrial outcomes, was an appreciation of the usability issues relating

Table 10.2 Tasks undertaken in the usability evaluation of PervaLaxis Touchscreen

Task 1 Videos	The user was required to open PervaLaxis Touchscreen, select a specific video about anaphylaxis and return to the tools menu
Task 2 Injector list	The user was required to use the injector expiry date tool in order to create a list of three specific adrenaline injector expiry dates (one non-expired, one expiring and one expired), delete one expiry date from the list and to edit another
Task 3 Trainer	The user was asked to open the trainer tool, run the injection demonstration steps and practise injecting adrenaline with the injector trainer
Task 4 Emergency action simulation	The user was required to press the emergency support button, watch an adrenaline injection video and simulate an injection using the injector trainer device

the use of ambient intelligence technology. Though, of course, the aim was not to supplant the traditional system, but rather to supplement it. For example, it was not anticipated that a mobile phone solution would replace the in-person clinical advice and training that forms the basis of the traditional system.

A usability study was undertaken at the University of Birmingham with 32 participants aged 18 to 40 years old. While testing with healthy volunteers is appropriate for preclinical testing, and there is the further issue that the vast majority of anaphylactic people are still preteen minors, the opinions of test volunteers with allergy experience was of interest. For this reason volunteers were asked about their allergy experience and the group of 32 constituted 16 people without allergies and 16 people with experience of allergies, i.e., were allergy sufferers themselves or caregivers of a person with allergies. The reported allergies ranged from mild to significant but no participants were carriers of adrenaline injectors. All 32 followed the same test procedure but, for interest only, the results of those who had experience of allergy were compared to those who had no experience.

Participants were provided with an explanation about anaphylaxis and adrenaline injections and were provided with documents on which this explanation was based. These documents are typical of the traditional system and included a manufacturer's injector information leaflet showing how to inject adrenaline and two information leaflets produced by the Anaphylaxis Campaign UK about anaphylaxis, its causes, symptoms, treatment and emergency recommendations. After consulting the documents, participants completed a system usability scale questionnaire [41]. They were then required to carry out four tasks (Table 10.2) using PervaLaxis Touchscreen. After finishing each task, they completed a NASA TLX workload questionnaire [42] and at the end of the evaluation they completed a system usability scale questionnaire for the mobile solution.

The SUS questionnaire was used to provide a measure of perceived usability, covering aspects of acceptance, need for support, training and system complexity [43, 44]. NASA TLX questionnaires were used to quantify levels of mental, physical and temporal demands, and self-reported levels of performance, effort and frustration.

Low demand levels could indicate that a task would be more likely to be successful in a real scenario [45]. ISO 9241-11 (Ergonomic of human system interaction—Part 11: Guidance on usability) [46] was used to measure effectiveness, efficiency, and satisfaction.

During the Pervalaxis tasks, participants could request assistance at any time. The number of requests was counted by the researcher. All requests were simple navigation queries. User keystrokes were automatically counted and logged by the system, and the task time was measured.

While undertaking the tasks, participants were encouraged to "think aloud" about their interaction with the system. They were particularly encouraged to make suggestions and to identify usability issues. All comments were recorded. Additional comments and suggestions were obtained from the completed workload and usability questionnaires and in a debrief talk.

A Shapiro-Wilk test was used to test if results were samples of a normally distributed population (Significance level = 0.05) [47]. Parametric t-tests were used on normally distributed results; and Mann-Whitney and Friedman Rank tests for results not normally distributed. The statistical tests were undertaken using SPSS® version 17.

10.5 Usability Results

10.5.1 System Usability Scale Results

Figure 10.6 shows the results of the system usability scale. These results revealed significant differences between PervaLaxis Touchscreen and the traditional system for all 10 questions in a 'holistic' approach. Here references to the traditional system mean the traditional system *alone*, i.e., the initial in-person advice and training and provision of hardcopy documentation that constitute the traditional system. References to PervaLaxis mean the PervaLaxis Touchscreen prototype supplementing the traditional system. Participants rated PervaLaxis better than the traditional system when they were asked whether they thought that they would like to use the system frequently. They found the traditional system more complex, more difficult to use, and less consistent and less integrated than PervaLaxis Touchscreen. They felt more confident using PervaLaxis Touchscreen and felt they needed to learn less to get going with it.

There were no significant differences between the results of allergic and non-allergic participants, with the exception of questions 4 and 10 where non-allergic participants reported more difficulty with the traditional system which, given their lack of allergy background, might be anticipated.

Table 10.3 shows the overall SUS score results and their meaning [48]. Unlike the traditional system that had a not acceptable score (between poor and OK), PervaLaxis Touchscreen score was acceptable (between good and excellent).

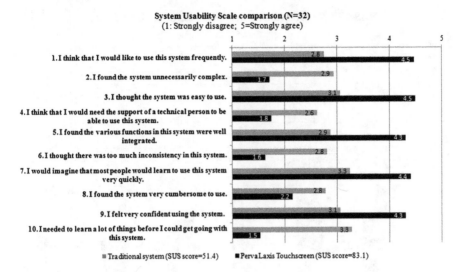

Fig. 10.6   System usability scale comparison between the traditional system and PervaLaxis Touchscreen and (N = 32, there were significant differences in all the SUS questions, p < 0.05)

Table 10.3   System usability scale results

System	Overall SUS score ±1 standard deviation (N = 32)	SUS meaning [48]
Traditional (document-based)	51.4 ± 19	Not acceptable (poor-ok SUS score)
PervaLaxis Touchscreen	83.1 ± 11	Acceptable (good-excellent SUS score)

10.5.2 Workload Results

Figure 10.7 shows the mental, physical and temporal demands, and the self-reported levels of performance, effort and frustration, quantified using the NASA TLX scales [42]. There were no significant differences between allergic and non-allergic participant results. Significant differences were found in the different scales for each task, as might be anticipated due to difference in keystrokes and actions required of each. But, although the time to complete each task was different, there were no significant differences in the temporal demand, suggesting participants felt no difference in time pressure.

Creating a list of injectors had a higher mental demand in comparison with using the emergency support button. Significant differences in physical demand $[X^2(3) = 31.39, p < 0.05]$ were shown for different tasks, with the injection trainer and emergency action simulation tasks requiring the greatest demand. Both these tasks required participants to simulate an injection. Furthermore, significant differences in performance $[X^2(3) = 13.9, p < 0.05]$, effort $[X^2(3) = 22.46, p < 0.05]$ and

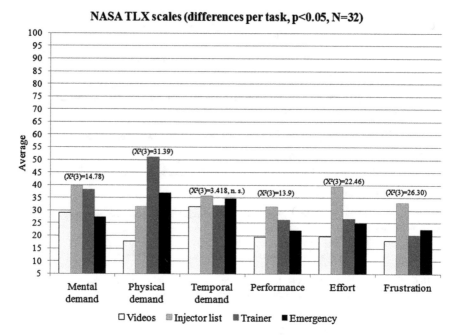

Fig. 10.7 NASA TLX scales results

frustration [$X^2(3) = 26.3$, p < 0.05], indicated that using the videos was an unde-manding task, but creating an injectors expiry date list was much more demanding. The injector list task had the highest demand in four out of six TLX scales.

10.5.3 Results from ISO 9241-11 Usability Measures

The Mann-Whitney test showed, again, that there was no significant difference between allergic and non-allergic participants using PervaLaxis Touchscreen in the ISO 9241-11 measures of effectiveness, efficiency, satisfaction and the amount of help provided to them. While satisfaction of allergic participants might have been expected to be higher than non-allergic participants, the satisfaction was high for both.

The Friedman Rank test revealed significant differences between the effectiveness, efficiency and number of requests for assistance for tasks (Fig. 10.8). For example, it can be seen in Fig. 10.8 that for task 1, using videos about anaphylaxis information, participants had significantly better effectiveness, better efficiency and asked for less help. This would mean that participants made less keystroke errors (i.e., were closer to the optimal number of keystrokes) and carried out this task quicker than the other tasks. In contrast, it is noticeable that the creation and editing of an injector

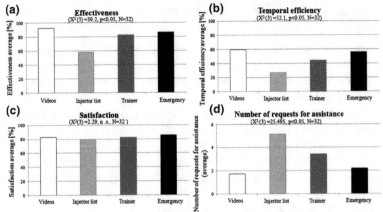

Note:
The X² indicates significant differences within tasks (figures a,b and d) or non-significant differences (figure c).

Usability measures, considering all parrticipants combined (as there was not siginificant differences between groups):

(a) Effectiveness: Accuracy and completeness with which users achieve specified goals.
   Effectiveness = (Correct number of keystrokes / participant's number of keystrokes) *100 [%] (Range: 0 to 100) ;

   Where: The correct (i.e., optimal) number of keystrokes are: {Videos= 4; Injector list= 44; Trainer=13;Emergency button=4}

(b) Efficiency: Resources expended in relation to the effectiveness with which users achieve goals, in this case time.

   Temporal efficiency = Effectiveness * $[(\dfrac{N * Optimal\ time}{\sum_{i=1}^{N} t_i})]$ [%] (Range: 0 to 100)

   Where: N:number of participants=32;   Optimal time=Expert's time; t_i:Time of participant i.

(c) Satisfaction: Freedom from discomfort, and positive attitudes towards the use of the application.
   Satisfaction with the implemented tools= (Subjective value) [%] (Range: 0:Very unlikely to 100:Very likely);

Statements asked to participants about satisfaction with the implemented tools

-Videos: I think this tool could help people learn about the anaphylactic condition.

-Injector list:I think this tool could help people manage their adrenaline injectors.

-Trainer: I think this tool could train people using the adrenaline injector.

-Emergency action simulation: I think this tool could help people to react correctly in an emergency event.

(d) The **number of requests for assistance** was quantified by the researcher. They were the number of times the participant received
   navigation advice per task.

Fig. 10.8 a–c Measures of usability according to ISO 9241 part 11. **d** Amount of navigation
assistance provided to participants

list produced on average more keystrokes than the optimal number, needed more
time to complete and required more navigation advice in comparison with the other
tasks. The test also suggested that the perceived satisfaction was not significantly
different within tasks with a visible average level around 80 %. This would indicate
that participants were satisfied with the implemented functionalities.

10.5.4 Observations and Comment Analysis

A content analysis was performed on the 257 comments collated from participants "think aloud" commentary, questionnaire submissions and debrief. These were categorized according to their respective task and identified as one of the following: (1) positive statements about PervaLaxis Touchscreen; or comments or suggestions regarding (2) the user interface; (3) the hardware and (4) the Smartphone processing speed. A trained independent coder carried a categorization. The reliability between coders had a satisfactory Cohen's kappa coefficient above 0.7.

Positive statements comprised 25 % of the total. Participants reported that PervaLaxis Touchscreen was interesting, useful for allergy management, preferable to the documents of the traditional system and that the information and functions were more accessible by being integrated in the mobile phone.

Thirty-four percentage of the total comments provided suggestions related to the user interface and 33 % related to functionality. Seven percentage commented on processing speed of the Smartphone. Participants commented on font size and colors, suggesting larger fonts and higher contrast colors, and suggested subtitles for the videos. Comments reflected that the Smartphone navigation was initially demanding but soon became easier.

The injector list task had positive reactions in, for example, the use of emoticons to provide a simple indicator of injector expiry date (a happy face for each in-date injector and a sad face for an out-of-date injector). The emergency support button received positive comments. Participants liked the possibility of sending the SMS messages with a single button press, including the name, GPS location and event. Their suggestions included provision for recorded voice messages and that the emergency function might also involve making a phone call after sending the SMS message.

In recording results of participants' injection attempts, we observed errors (deviations from the information and instructions provided) in injection site, not applying sufficient force, not holding the injector in place for 10 seconds and not massaging the injection site. It was interesting to observe a reduction in these errors on the subsequent injection required in task 4 (emergency action simulation), suggesting that practice and feedback from PervaLaxis might help users improve performance. For example, in the first injection in task 3, two participants held the injector the wrong way around and would have injected their own thumbs if the trainer had been a real injector. There were no such errors in the subsequent injection. Similarly, 4 participants failed to hold the injector trainer in place for 10 s after the first injection, but all performed correctly on the next injection. However, there were 5 in 32 attempts in task 4 which failed to make sufficient force to make the correct "jab" type injection motion.

The injector trainer testing demonstrated that the simple thresholding detection method was limited. For example, only 20 (out of 32) of the injection attempts were correctly detected on the first occasion (task 3); and 25 out of 32 in the second occasion (task 4), with only five potentially accounted for by user error. An improved method of detection would not only improve reporting of possible injections but would reduce the possibility of false positive events.

10.6 Conclusions and Further Work

This chapter explored allergy management and the requirements of people affected by anaphylactic allergy and presented the usability evaluation of PervaLaxis Touchscreen, a prototype system designed to support people managing allergies.

Test results suggest that wireless ambient intelligence technology, in the form of a Smartphone and accelerometer has the potential to provide usable support for anaphylaxis management. Results showed that the PervaLaxis Touchscreen prototype, supplementing basic anaphylaxis training with the traditional system, was preferable to the traditional document-based system alone. Participants reported that PervaLaxis Touchscreen was interesting, useful for allergy management, preferable to the documents of the traditional system and that the information and functions were more accessible by being integrated in the mobile phone.

Because allergic people and their carers normally carry adrenaline injectors and mobile phones (increasingly Smartphones with in-built GPS) the system would require little in the way of technology imposition for implementation while providing functionality not available elsewhere. There are, however, inherent issues associated with SMS message reliability, mobile phone coverage and the development of the wider infrastructure to support messaging that would benefit further consideration. Further work on injection detection would also be useful for improving sensing accuracy and further consideration of a system of messaging could benefit personalization and flexibility.

Although positive feedback was received about the potential of the emergency support function, since a real anaphylactic event is neither ethically possible nor desirable [49], evaluation is necessarily limited to a simulated scenario in a controlled setting. However, it is hoped that this research could lead to further studies in the support of allergy management and inform work leading to clinical trials.

Acknowledgments We would like to thank the University of Birmingham, CONACyT, The Anaphylaxis Campaign UK, Cadbury Schweppes Foundation, SEP, our allergic and non-allergic participants, Dr. Tim Collins and the System Usability Scale creators. We would also like to thank the editor, our reviewers and the proof readers of this chapter for their very valuable feedback.

References

1. L. U. Hernandez-Munoz and S. I. Woolley. A personal handheld device to support people with life-threatening anaphylactic allergies (PervaLaxis). International Journal of Handheld Computing Research. IGI; 2010 Jan 1; 1(1):64–78.

170 L. U. Hernandez-Munoz and S. I. Woolley

2. H. Sampson, A. Munoz-Furlong, R. Campbell R, et al. Second Symposium on the Definition and Management of Anaphylaxis: Summary report - Second National Institute of Allergy and Infectious Disease/Food Allergy and Anaphylaxis Network Symposium. Annals of emergency medicine. 2006; 47(4):373–80.
3. Allergy UK. 2011. Available from:http://www.allergyuk.org/
4. The anaphylaxis Campaign UK. 2010. Available from: www.anaphylaxis.org.uk.
5. The World Allergic Organization. Anaphylaxis: Synopsis. 2006. Retrieved on: 2012 Apr 21. Available from: http://www.worldallergy.org/professional/allergic_diseases_center/anaphylaxis/anaphylaxissynopsis.php
6. F. Simons and H. Sampson. Anaphylaxis epidemic: fact or fiction? The Journal of allergy and clinical immunology. Elsevier Ltd; 2008 Dec.; 122(6):1166–8.
7. A. Sherwood, Allergy-free Cookbook. London, UK. Dorling Kindersley Limited.; 2007.
8. Y. S. Xu, S. B. Waserman, S. Waserman, et al. Food allergy management from the perspective of patients or caregivers, and allergists: a qualitative study. Allergy, asthma, and clinical immunology: official journal of the Canadian Society of Allergy and Clinical Immunology
9. S. H. Sicherer, J. A. Forman and S.A. Noone. Use Assessment of Self-Administered Epinephrine Among Food-Allergic Children and Pediatricians. Pediatrics. American Academy of Pediatrics; 2000; 105(2), pp. 359–62.
10. K. Carlisle, P. Vargas, S. Noone, et al. Food allergy education for school nurses: a needs assessment survey by the consortium of food allergy research. The Journal of school nursing: the official publication of the National Association of School Nurses [Internet]. 2010 Oct.
11. R. Pumphrey. Anaphylaxis: can we tell who is at risk of a fatal reaction? Current opinion in allergy and clinical immunology. 2004 Aug; 4(4):285–90.
12. M. A. Warner, C. D. Crisci, S. Del Giacco, et al. Allergy Practice Worldwide: A Report by the World Allergy Organization Specialty and Training Council. Journal of the World Allergy Organization. 2006; 18(1):4–10.
13. M. Kastner, L. Harada and S. Waserman. Gaps in anaphylaxis management at the level of physicians, patients, and the community: a systematic review of the literature. Allergy. John Wiley & Sons A/S; 2010; 65(4):435–44.
14. H. Blake. Innovation in practice: mobile phone technology in patient care. British journal of community nursing. 2008 Apr; 13(4):160, 162–5.
15. R. Ballagas, J. Borchers, M. Rohs, et al. The Smart Phone: A Ubiquitous Input Device. IEEE Pervasive Computing. 2006; 5(1):70–7.
16. K. Yamauchi, W. Chen and D. Wei. 3G mobile phone applications in telemedicine - a survey. Computer and Information Technology, 2005. CIT 2005. The Fifth International Conference on. 2005. page 956–60.
17. M. Boulos, S. Wheeler, C. Tavares and R. Jones. How smartphones are changing the face of mobile and participatory healthcare: an overview, with example from eCAALYX. Biomedical engineering online.
18. P. Yu and H. Yu. Lessons learned from the practice of mobile health application development. Computer Software and Applications Conference, 2004. COMPSAC 2004. Proceedings of the 28th Annual International. 2004. page 58–9.
19. CardioTrainer. Android Market. 2010. Retrieved on: 2010 Sep 24. Available from: http://www.android.com/market/#app=com.wsl.CardioTrainer
20. Instant heart rate. appbrain.com. 2010. Retrieved on: 2010 Sep 28. Available from: http://www.appbrain.com/app/si.modula.android.instantheartrate
21. eDiabetes. Android Market. 2010. Retrieved on: 2010 Sep 24. Available from: http://www.android.com/market/#app=com.physiosensing.eDiabetes_Pro
22. HandyLogs sugar. App Store. 2010. Retrieved on: 2010 Sep 28. Available from: http://www.apple.com/webapps/utilities/handylogssugar.html
23. Diet & Food Tracker. Android Market. 2010. Retrieved on: 2010 Sep 24. Available from: http://www.android.com/market/#app=com.sparkpeople.app
24. Medlife. App Store. 2010. Retrieved on: 2010 Sep 30. Available from: http://www.apple.com/webapps/utilities/medfile.html

25. MobileCoach. Windows market place. 2010. Retrieved on: 2010 Sep 28]. Available from: http://marketplace.windowsphone.com/details.aspx?appId=72ab7593-9a55-434f-b427-7f9c317cd47b&retURL=/search.aspx?keywords=health

26. E. J. Gómez, M. E. Hernando Pérez, T. Vering, et al. The INCA system: a further step towards a telemedical artificial pancreas. IEEE transactions on information technology in biomedicine. 2008 Jul; 12(4):470–9.

27. S. Phan, D. Shen and A. Asbeck. Discreet, Painless Glucose Monitoring with your Mobile Phone. Mobile phone implantable monitor interface. 2010. Retrieved on: 2010 Sep 30. Available from: http://www.scribd.com/doc/14848043/Mobile-Phone-Implantable-Monitor-Interface

28. L. Yung-Hsiu, S. Guo, C. Rong-Rong and C. Her-Kun. Developing diabetes self-care supporting service: A systemic approach. 2009 IEEE International Conference on Service-Oriented Computing and Applications (SOCA). IEEE; 2009 Dec; 00(c):1–7.

29. C. H. Salvador, M. P. Carrasco, M. De Mingo, et al. Airmed-cardio: a GSM and Internet services-based system for out-of-hospital follow-up of cardiac patients. IEEE transactions on Information Technology in Biomedicine. 2005 Mar; 9(1):73–85.

30. T. Markow, N. Ramakrishnan, K. Huang, et al. Mobile Music Touch: Vibration stimulus in hand rehabilitation. 4th International Conference on Pervasive Computing Technologies for Healthcare (PervasiveHealth), 2010. 2010. page 1–8.

31. N. Nasr, S. Torsi, S. Mawson, et al. Self management of stroke supported by assistive technology. 2009 Virtual Rehabilitation International Conference. IEEE; 2009 Jun; 6:193–193.

32. G. Vavoula and P. Lonsdale. Mobile learning for young allergy sufferers: A report exploring research opportunities, challenges, methods and best practices. 2007 Jan.

33. K. Gassner, B. Vollmer, M. Prehn, et al. Smart food: mobile guidance for food-allergic people. Seventh IEEE International Conference on E-Commerce Technology, 2005. CEC 2005. 2005. page 531–4.

34. E. Badinelli. Scanavert: detection and alarm against ingredient harm. CCNC 2006. 2006 3rd IEEE Consumer Communications and Networking Conference, 2006. IEEE; 2006; 2:1286–7.

35. A. J. Jara, M. Zamora and A. Skarmeta. Drug identification and interaction checker based on IoT to minimize adverse drug reactions and improve drug compliance. Personal and Ubiquitous Computing. 2012 Oct 31.

36. Immunology. App Store. 2010. Retrieved on: 2010 Sep 28. Available from: http://www.apple.com/webapps/news/allergyimmunologyheadlinenews.html

37. Allergy Free Passport. 2010. Retrieved on: 2010 Sep 24. Available from: http://allergyfreepassport.com/mobile-apps/

38. L. Duffett-leger and J. Lumsden. Interactive Online Health Promotion Interventions: A " Health Check ". 2008.

39. UK Government, Communication providers, The Emergency Services, Ofcom, Action on Hearing Loss. emergencySMS. 2012. Retrieved on: 2012 Dec 1. Available from: http://www.emergencysms.org.uk

40. N. McAllister. US text-to-911 emergency SMS to go live by 2014. The register. 2012. Retrieved on: 2013 Jan 5. Available from:http://www.theregister.co.uk/2012/12/07/us_text_to_911_emergency_rollout/

41. J. Brooke. System Usability Scale [Internet]. Usabilitynet.org. 2006. Retrieved on: 2006 Jun 1. Available from: www.usabilitynet.org/trump/documents/Suschapt.doc

42. NASA. NASA TLX: Task Load Index. 2003. Available from: http://humansystems.arc.nasa.gov/groups/TLX/

43. M. Jones and G. Marsden. Mobile Interaction Design. London: John Wiley & Sons, Ltd; 2006.

44. J. Preece, Y. Rogers and H. Sharp. Interaction design, beyond human-computer interaction. New York: Wiley & Sons, Inc.; 2002.

45. S. Brewster, J. Lumsden, M. Bell, M. Hall and S.Tasker S. Multimodal " Eyes-Free " Interaction Techniques for Wearable Devices. Computer Human-Interaction CHI. 2003.

46. ISO 9241–11. Ergonomic requirements for office work with visual display terminal (VDTs) - Part 11: Guidance on usability. 1998.

47. A. Field. Discovering statistics using SPSS for Windows. London: SAGE Publications Ltd; 2000.
48. A. Bangor, P. T. Kortum and J.T. Miller. An Empirical Evaluation of the System Usability Scale. International Journal of Human-Computer Interaction. 2008 Jul 29; 24(6):574–94.
49. R. S. Pumphrey. Lessons for management of anaphylaxis from a study of fatal reactions. Clinical and experimental allergy: journal of the British Society for Allergy and, Clinical Immunology. 2000 Aug, 30(8): 1144–50.

GPSR Compliance
The European Union's (EU) General Product Safety Regulation (GPSR) is a set
of rules that requires consumer products to be safe and our obligations to
ensure this.

If you have any concerns about our products, you can contact us on

ProductSafety@springernature.com

In case Publisher is established outside the EU, the EU authorized
representative is:

Springer Nature Customer Service Center GmbH
Europaplatz 3
69115 Heidelberg, Germany